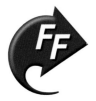

Fast Facts:
Diabetes Mellitus

Fourth edition

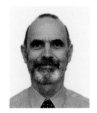

Ian N Scobie MD FRCP
Consultant Endocrinologist
Medway Maritime Hospital
Gillingham, Kent, and
Honorary Senior Lecturer
King's College London School of Medicine
London, UK

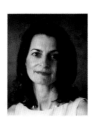

Katherine Samaras MBBS PHD FRACP
Associate Professor
The University of New South Wales, and
Senior Staff Specialist, St Vincent's Hospital, and
Head, Dia
Garvan In
Darlinghu

D1334259

Declaration of Independence
This book is as balanced and as practical as we can make it.
Ideas for improvement are always welcome: feedback@fastfacts.com

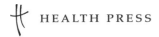

HEALTH PRESS

Fast Facts: Diabetes Mellitus
First published 1996; second edition 2001; third edition 2009;
reprinted 2010
Fourth edition June 2012

Text © 2012 Ian N Scobie, Katherine Samaras
© 2012 in this edition Health Press Limited
Health Press Limited, Elizabeth House, Queen Street, Abingdon,
Oxford OX14 3LN, UK
Tel: +44 (0)1235 523233
Fax: +44 (0)1235 523238

Book orders can be placed by telephone or via the website.
For regional distributors or to order via the website, please go to:
fastfacts.com

For telephone orders, please call +44 (0)1752 202301 (UK, Europe and Asia–
Pacific), 1 800 247 6553 (USA, toll free) or +1 419 281 1802 (Americas).

Fast Facts is a trademark of Health Press Limited.

A CIP record for this title is available from the British Library.

ISBN 978-1-908541-14-7

Scobie IN (Ian)
Fast Facts: Diabetes Mellitus/
Ian N Scobie, Katherine Samaras

Medical illustrations by Dee McLean, London, UK.
Typesetting and page layout by Zed, Oxford, UK.
Printed by Latimer Trend & Company Limited, Plymouth, UK.

Text printed on biodegradable and recyclable paper manufactured
using elemental chlorine free (ECF) wood pulp from well-
managed forests.

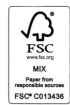

FSC
www.fsc.org
MIX
Paper from
responsible sources
FSC® C013436

Introduction

National data demonstrate an alarming increase in the prevalence of diabetes mellitus in the developed world. The 2011 National Diabetes Fact Sheet in the USA tells us that the prevalence of diabetes is 8.3% in the US population, varying from 7.1% in non-Hispanic whites to 12.6% in non-Hispanic blacks (with even higher rates in Mexican Americans). This equates to 18.8 million people with diabetes (and 7.0 million with undiagnosed diabetes). Data from the UK Quality and Outcomes Framework reveal that 4.26% of the UK population has diabetes, equating to 2.8 million people. The number of people with diabetes worldwide projected for 2025 is more than 300 million.

With increasing urbanization in India there has been an explosive increase in the prevalence of diabetes, which has now reached 8.0%, with 50 million people with type 2 diabetes. In China, diabetes has become a major public health problem, with an estimated prevalence of 9.7%. Although the incidence of new cases of type 1 diabetes is increasing in many countries, the increase in new cases of type 2 diabetes is of near-epidemic proportions. Societal factors seem to be the likely culprits behind this massive increase in diabetes prevalence in both developed and developing countries. Such factors include the adoption of a westernized diet and lifestyle and a decline in physical activity leading to ever-rising rates of obesity. In the developing world, population movements from rural agricultural areas to urban areas are associated with the acquisition of type 2 diabetes.

Cardiovascular disease remains a significant cause of death in both type 1 and type 2 diabetes. Preventive strategies are needed to minimize cardiovascular risk and improve outcome. However, these should not be at the expense of the pursuit of good blood glucose control, as this closely correlates with the development of those specific microvascular complications of diabetes that so clearly define this ubiquitous condition.

In parallel with the increase in diabetes prevalence, diabetes research continues to flourish; from basic science through to randomized prospective clinical trials, there is a great endeavor to determine the exact pathogenesis of type 1 diabetes, type 2 diabetes and other forms of diabetes and their complications, and to understand how best to prevent and treat them. One particular feature has been the recent advent of new pharmaceutical products to treat type 2 diabetes, albeit associated with problems along the way. Research continues into the development of a possible vaccine to prevent type 1 diabetes.

The aim of this fourth edition of *Fast Facts: Diabetes Mellitus* is to provide readers with an up-to-date picture of our understanding of diabetes mellitus and its various causes, its clinical manifestations and the treatment strategies that can be used to reduce the burden of its metabolic consequences.

The prevalence of diabetes around the world is increasing rapidly (see the Introduction). Of the seven regions monitored by the International Diabetes Federation (IDF) around the world, the North America/ Caribbean region has the highest national prevalence (11.7% in 2011), followed by the Middle East and North Africa (9.1%). Worldwide comparative prevalence of diabetes is shown in Figure 1.1.

It is clear some nations have substantially higher rates of diabetes. Data from 2011 in the *Diabetes Atlas* of the IDF show the highest national prevalence of diabetes in adults from Kiribati, the Marshall islands, Nauru, Lebanon and other Middle Eastern nations (Table 1.1).

Mortality

Diabetes caused 4.6 million deaths globally in 2011 – approximately 6% of the total world mortality. Even more people have died from cardiovascular disease, the risk of which is increased by diabetes-

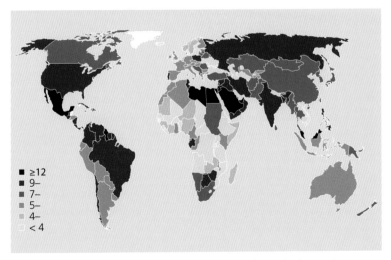

Figure 1.1 Comparative prevalence of diabetes: the scale shows the percentage of the adult population affected by diabetes. *IDF Diabetes Atlas*, fifth edition. © International Diabetes Federation, 2011.

TABLE 1.1

Countries with the highest comparative prevalence of diabetes in adults aged 20–79 years

Country	Prevalence (%)
Kiribati	25.7
Marshall islands	22.2
Kuwait	21.1
Nauru	20.7
Lebanon	20.2
Qatar	20.2
Saudi Arabia	20.0
Bahrain	19.9
Tuvalu	19.5
United Arab Emirates	19.2

Data from *IDF Diabetes Atlas*, fifth edition. © International Diabetes Federation, 2011.

related comorbidities such as hyperlipidemia, hypertension and renal disease. Data for deaths attributable to diabetes according to world regions are shown in Figure 1.2.

Indirect burden

Globally, the greatest number of people with diabetes are in the age range 40–59 years, a time in which productivity at work and contribution to family life is anticipated. Illness, disability and premature death in this age group profoundly affect personal and family life, communities and national productivity. IDF data show that preventable complications of diabetes account for an additional 23 million years of life lost through disability and reduced quality of life.

Predicted picture

Data extrapolations suggest the prevalence will continue to rise steeply and that by 2030, 552 million people will be affected. The IDF has

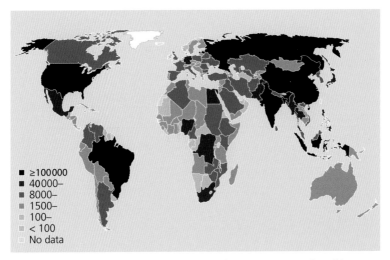

Figure 1.2 Worldwide deaths in adults aged 20–79 years attributable to diabetes in 2011. *IDF Diabetes Atlas*, fifth edition. © International Diabetes Federation, 2011.

identified several reasons for the steep increase anticipated in diabetes prevalence: overweight and obesity, unhealthy eating, sedentary lifestyles, urbanization and an aging population.

Asia

In terms of the population-based burden of diabetes, China has the highest number of people affected, based on 2011 data collected by the IDF, followed by India and the USA (Table 1.2). Rapid changes in lifestyle associated with westernization have led to rapid increases in prevalence of diabetes throughout Asia. Of concern, recent data show no sign that the rate is slowing. People of Asian descent develop diabetes at lower degrees of obesity and at younger ages. There are also data to suggest Asian people suffer longer from diabetes complications and die earlier than people in other regions. An accelerating factor appears to be childhood obesity, which is increasing at alarming rates in Asia.

Access to drugs

There are clear disparities between nations in access to drugs. About 80% of people with diabetes live in the world's poorest nations, but

TABLE 1.2

Countries with the highest numbers of adults (20–79 years) with diabetes

Country	Number affected (millions)
People's Republic of China	90.0
India	61.3
USA	23.7
Russia	12.6
Brazil	12.4
Japan	10.7
Mexico	10.3
Bangladesh	8.4
Egypt	7.3
Indonesia	7.3

Data from *IDF Diabetes Atlas*, fifth edition. © International Diabetes Federation, 2011.

80% of medical expenditure for diabetes occurs in the world's economically richest nations. Insulin is not available in many such areas because of its cost. Inevitably, people with type 1 diabetes who cannot access insulin die.

Recent trends in children

Type 1 diabetes develops in about 70,000 children under the age of 14 every year. Recent data indicate the rate of new cases of type 1 diabetes is increasing by 3% every year, promoted by, among other factors, escalating rates of childhood obesity. About 25% of all cases of type 1 diabetes are in South East Asia, with about 20% in Europe. Finland, Sweden and Norway have the highest incidence of type 1 diabetes. The rate of type 2 diabetes is also increasing in children.

Key points – epidemiology

- The prevalence of diabetes is increasing around the world, reflecting the massive societal changes in dietary habits, with energy overconsumption, an increase in sedentary lifestyle and obesity.
- Different ethnic groups are particularly susceptible to diabetes.
- The obesity epidemic is impacting on earlier development of both type 1 and type 2 diabetes.
- The impact of diabetes and its complications will have the greatest burden on resource-poor nations with limited access to insulin and renal replacement (dialysis and transplantation).

Key references

International Diabetes Federation. *Diabetes Atlas*, 5th edn. IDF, Brussels, 2011. Available from www.idf.org/atlasmap/atlasmap, last accessed 8 May 2012.

Yoon KH, Lee JH, Kim JW et al. Epidemic obesity and type 2 diabetes in Asia. *Lancet* 2006;368:1681–8.

Zimmet P, Alberti KG, Shaw J. Global and societal implications of the diabetes epidemic. *Nature* 2001;414:782–7.

Early detection of diabetes is critical, as appropriate treatment will prevent the complications of diabetes and the significant burden this places on an individual's quality of life, morbidity and mortality. Early detection of impaired fasting glucose or impaired glucose tolerance allows early intervention with appropriate lifestyle change and can defer and even prevent the onset of diabetes. Thus, early detection plays an important role in optimizing health.

The diagnosis of diabetes has changed progressively over the last couple of decades; criteria have become simplified and now recognize that diabetic complications occur with glucose levels previously considered normal. Diagnostic criteria are likely to change again in the future.

The current diagnostic cut-offs are listed in Table 2.1 and reflect the American Diabetes Association (ADA) guidelines of 2011. Fasting

TABLE 2.1

Diagnostic cut-offs for disorders of glucose metabolism

Method	Fasting glucose		2-hour glucose	
	mmol/L	mg/dL	mmol/L	mg/dL
Fasting glucose*				
Normal	< 5.6	< 100		
Impaired fasting glucose	5.6–6.9	100–125		
Diabetes	≥ 7.0	≥ 126		
75 g oral glucose tolerance test				
Normal			< 7.8	< 140
Impaired glucose tolerance			7.8–11.1	140–199
Diabetes			> 11.1	> 200

American Diabetes Association 2011.
*Fasting: 8 hours or no energy intake.

glucose ≥ 7.0 mmol/L (126 mg/dL) is generally diagnostic of diabetes mellitus. Random glucose > 11.1 mmol/L (200 mg/dL) is also diagnostic in a patient with polyuria, polydipsia or unexplained weight loss.

These cut-offs establish the diagnosis of diabetes, after which it is left to the clinician to consider and determine the cause or type of diabetes. This can be determined on clinical findings and, if required, other investigations or antibody testing. Further characterization of diabetes types is discussed below.

Glucose tolerance testing

Glucose tolerance should be formally tested when glucose levels fall short of diagnostic cut-offs and the patient is considered 'at-risk' (Table 2.2).

A glucose tolerance test focuses on the 2-hour glucose response following a 75 g oral glucose load. The glucose load is given as a drink. Cut-offs are given in Table 2.1: essentially a 2-hour glucose response > 11.1 mmol/L (200 mg/dL) is diagnostic of diabetes and < 7.8 mmol/L (140 mg/dL) considered normal. The intermediate range in 2-hour glucose response is called 'impaired glucose tolerance'.

TABLE 2.2

At-risk patients to consider for screening for diabetes

- Overweight or obese
- Past history of gestational diabetes
- First-degree relative(s) with diabetes
- Hepatitis C infection
- Predisposed ethnic groups, including people from the Middle Eastern nations
- Chronic corticosteroid therapy
- Solid organ transplant recipients
- HIV-infected recipients of combined antiretroviral therapy
- Cystic fibrosis
- Lipodystrophy (congenital or acquired)

The glucose tolerance test is a useful provocation test that can be used for early detection of diabetes in the at-risk patient (see Table 2.2). It is also diagnostically useful in women with impaired fasting glucose (fasting glucose 5.6–6.9 mmol/L [100–125 mg/dL]), for whom the fasting glucose test is less sensitive for diabetes.

The current ADA criteria require confirmation by repeat testing on a subsequent day. This should be tempered by the clinical situation. For example, it would not be necessary to confirm in a young hyperglycemic patient with symptoms of hyperglycemia who has early ketoacidosis. Similarly, repeat testing is not appropriate for the unwell patient found to be hyperglycemic with sepsis, acute infection or acute myocardial infarction, or post-transplantation, for whom treatment of both the acute underlying illness and associated hyperglycemia is indicated.

Measurement of glycated hemoglobin (HbA_{1c}) is currently under consideration as a diabetes screening tool and it is likely it will be adopted. Current obstacles include determination of cut-offs, but also international standardization of the assay.

Special considerations in screening

In patients receiving corticosteroids, fasting glucose levels are often normal; steroid effects on glucose metabolism do not usually manifest till mid-afternoon. Therefore, in these patients, the best time to screen is with a random glucose level between 15:00 and 17:00 hours.

Impaired fasting glucose

It is now recognized that a fasting glucose level between 5.6 and 6.9 mmol/L (100–125 mg/dL) is 'prediabetic'. Studies show these individuals are already developing diabetic complications such as microalbuminuria and are at increased cardiovascular risk. Thus, early detection is important for early intervention for complication development. Further, there is increasing evidence that the β cell dysfunction in prediabetes may be impacted by early lifestyle intervention, such that progression of the β cell secretory impairment might be slowed.

Determination of type

In those diagnosed with diabetes, it is important to distinguish between the different types. This is simple in those cases of lean children, adolescents or adults who present with sudden onset of polyuria and polydipsia, who clearly have type 1 diabetes. Similarly, it may be relatively clear cut in the obese middle-aged person with multiple family members who have lifestyle- or tablet-managed type 2 diabetes. It can be less clear cut in some situations, however.

Latent autoimmune diabetes in adults (LADA) provides a good example. It may appear identical to type 2 diabetes but be difficult to manage with standard oral medications, with patients progressing to insulin therapy. Recent studies show that early instigation of insulin therapy in this diabetes subgroup is associated with better glycemic control than use of sulfonylureas; a large randomized study is currently under way.

To distinguish LADA from type 2 diabetes, detection of serum autoimmune antibodies is useful, specifically glutamic acid decarboxylase (GAD) antibodies and cytoplasmic islet cell antibodies (ICA). Antibody testing should be considered if the individual with diabetes has any of the following features:

- lean
- other autoimmune conditions (primary hypothyroidism, Graves disease, celiac disease, premature ovarian failure, Addison's disease)
- strong family history of any autoimmune disease
- strong family history of diabetes without obesity for which insulin therapy was required.

While distinguishing LADA/type 1 from 'usual' type 2 diabetes is of significance for making therapeutic decisions, there are other types of diabetes for which choice of therapy may be influenced by the type of diabetes present. These are discussed in more detail in Chapter 7.

Underlying causes

It is also relevant to consider underlying causes of diabetes, such as hemochromatosis and rare endocrinopathies, such as Cushing's syndrome and acromegaly. Seeking appropriate clinical signs is useful.

Hemochromatosis may be screened by serum ferritin levels. However, caution is needed in interpreting results in obese individuals with fatty liver disease, for whom ferritin is often raised. If suspected, formal endocrine consultation may be required to exclude Cushing's syndrome and acromegaly.

Key points – diagnosis

- Screening for diabetes should be undertaken annually with a fasting glucose level.
- Always consider diabetes mellitus in high-risk populations, including those with a family history, the obese, corticosteroid recipients and transplantation recipients.

Key references

American Diabetes Association. Diagnosis and classification of diabetes mellitus. *Diabetes Care* 2008;31(suppl 1):S55–60.

American Diabetes Association. Standards of care. Causes and diagnosis of diabetes mellitus. *Diabetes Care* 2011;34(suppl 1): S12–15.

3 Type 1 diabetes mellitus

Type 1 diabetes afflicts millions of people worldwide. Type 1a is characterized by the presence of autoantibodies that cause immune destruction of the β cells of the islets of Langerhans; in type 1b diabetes, such evidence is lacking. The hallmark of type 1 diabetes mellitus (also known, historically, as insulin-dependent diabetes mellitus) is insulin deficiency. Loss of normal insulin secretion from the endocrine pancreas is caused by progressive destruction of the β cells in the islets of Langerhans. The resulting lack of insulin production causes major abnormalities of carbohydrate, fat and protein metabolism, the most dramatic of which is hyperglycemia.

The classic symptoms of diabetes (Table 3.1) emerge when approximately 90% of the β cells in the islets have been destroyed. Although characteristically such symptoms have a relatively sudden onset, the initiating pathophysiological process leading to the clinical emergence of type 1 diabetes may occur over a prolonged period of time (Figure 3.1). Indeed, recent studies have suggested that, in some patients, residual insulin secretory capacity may be preserved for months or even, in a small proportion of cases, years.

Type 1 diabetes differs from type 2 in many ways; the key features of type 1 diabetes are illustrated in Table 3.2. In clinical practice it can sometimes be difficult to determine whether an individual patient has type 1 or type 2 diabetes when classic features are not present. Testing

TABLE 3.1

Classic symptoms of new-onset diabetes mellitus

- Thirst
- Polydipsia
- Polyuria
- Weight loss
- Pruritus vulvae
- Balanitis
- Blurred vision

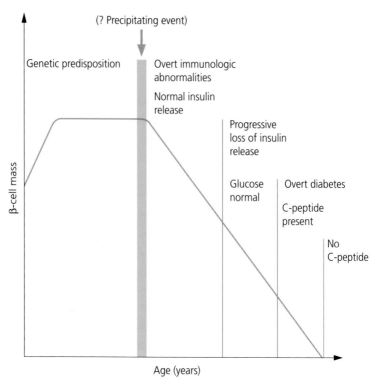

Figure 3.1 Stages in the development of type 1 diabetes.

TABLE 3.2

Key features of type 1 diabetes mellitus

- Insulin treatment is necessary to sustain life
- Patient is prone to ketosis and associated acidemia
- Relatively acute onset of disease
- Onset is most common in youth, but it may occur at any age
- Strong association with HLA haplotypes DR3 and DR4
- Presence of specific autoantibodies
- Positive family history in 10% of patients
- 30–50% concordance in identical twins

HLA, human leukocyte antigen.

for autoimmune markers of type 1 diabetes and insulin secretory reserve helps to distinguish the two conditions.

Although the precise cause or causes of type 1 diabetes remain to be elucidated, the best working model is that something in the environment triggers autoimmune damage in a person genetically prone to the disease (Figure 3.2). An increase in the incidence of cases of type 1 diabetes is being observed in many areas of the world. As this is unlikely to be related to a change in the gene pool, it suggests that some unidentified environmental factor or factors is triggering the increase. Children who develop type 1 diabetes are often heavier in early childhood and tend to be taller. Some have speculated that the increasing prevalence of obesity in childhood is the cause of the increasing incidence of type 1 diabetes (the 'accelerator hypothesis'), but this theory remains far from proven.

Environmental factors

Viral infection has long been considered the most likely environmental factor involved in type 1 diabetes. In humans, evidence comes from the observation that there are seasonal and geographic variations in the onset of the disease. Lower rates of incidence have been reported in the late spring and summer and higher rates in the winter in both

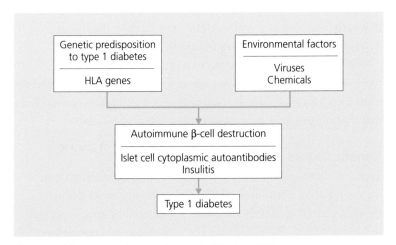

Figure 3.2 Proposed etiology of type 1 diabetes. HLA, human leukocyte antigen.

the northern and southern hemispheres. The age-related and seasonal incidence graphs show peaks that coincide with the age of maximum exposure to viral infections and with the time of year when such infections are more common in the general population.

Mumps and Coxsackie viruses may cause acute pancreatitis and Coxsackie virus infection may lead to inflammatory destruction of β cells. A significant association between enterovirus infection detected by molecular methods and autoimmune type 1 diabetes has been demonstrated. The precise temporal relationship remains to be elucidated. Coxsackie B viruses have been isolated from the pancreases of patients with new-onset type 1 diabetes. Viruses (such as Coxsackie) may directly attack the β cell or may act by initiating autoimmune destruction of the β cell. The only certain association is between rubella infection during pregnancy and increased risk of the neonate developing type 1 diabetes. Despite this and the longstanding suspicion of a relationship between type 1 diabetes and preceding viral infection, the precise role of viral infections in the etiology of type 1 diabetes is not yet clear.

Other agents. Bovine serum albumin has long been suggested as a cause of type 1 diabetes in children who may have had early exposure to cow's milk, but this theory remains unproven. Similarly, reports that early ingestion of cereal or gluten may increase the risk of development of type 1 diabetes remain to be substantiated.

Nitrosamines in smoked or cured meats may be diabetogenic. Furthermore, certain chemicals such as streptozotocin, alloxan and the rat poison Vacor are directly toxic to β cells, but it seems very unlikely that these agents have a significant role in causing the disease.

Genetic factors

Type 1 diabetes is a complex genetic trait. Multiple inherited genetic factors influence both susceptibility and resistance to the disease. Familial clustering of type 1 diabetes is suggested by an average risk in siblings of 6%, compared with 0.4% in the general population. The concordance for type 1 diabetes is approximately 30–50% for monozygotic or identical twins (who share 100% of their genes).

Nevertheless, a family history of type 1 diabetes is more likely to be absent than present in index cases.

Many studies have evaluated candidate genes for disease association, leading to the identification of two chromosomal regions with consistent and significant association with type 1 diabetes. These are the human leukocyte antigen (HLA) region and the insulin gene region.

The HLA region is a cluster of genes located within the major histocompatibility complex (MHC) on chromosome 6p21. Of these genes, it is estimated that the HLA region (designated the major locus of type 1 diabetes *IDDM1* [also known as *HLA-DQB1*]) accounts for up to 40–50% of the familial clustering of type 1 diabetes. HLA class II gene alleles are, statistically, the most strongly associated with type 1 diabetes, with good evidence that particular alleles of the *HLA-DQA1*, *-DQB1* (previously referred to as *HLA-DR3/4*) and *-DRB-1* loci are all primarily involved in the genetic predisposition to type 1 diabetes. Combinations of *HLA-DQ* genes and particularly those present in *HLA-DQ2/DQ8* heterozygotes are linked with disease susceptibility. Indeed, approximately 30% of patients with type 1 diabetes are *HLA-DQ2/DQ8* heterozygotes. Other *HLA-DQ* alleles, by contrast, confer disease protection.

Non-HLA-encoded susceptibility. Only one non-HLA gene has been generally accepted as a genetic contributor to type 1 diabetes risk, and that is the insulin gene (*INS*) region mapped to chromosome 11p15.5 that is now designated *IDDM2*. The insulin gene is a very plausible candidate susceptibility locus, as insulin may act as an autoantigen in the immune-mediated process leading to type 1 diabetes. Other susceptibility loci have been identified in certain groups of people with type 1 diabetes.

Mechanisms of autoimmune β cell destruction

While there is an abundant body of evidence to suggest an autoimmune pathogenesis for type 1 diabetes, there remains an incomplete understanding of the relationship between the described genetic susceptibility to the disorder and the observed abnormal immune response secondary to a putative environmental trigger. Examination of islets from pancreatic biopsy or at postmortem from patients with recently diagnosed type 1 diabetes shows a diffuse lymphocytic infiltration of the islets, a process known as insulitis (Figure 3.3). Insulitis is deemed to be the precursor of the process of progressive β cell destruction.

Autoantibodies

Islet cell antibodies (ICA) are present in the serum of approximately 75% of patients at the onset of type 1 diabetes (Figure 3.4). Islet cell constituent autoantibodies are present in 15–85% of patients around the time of disease presentation and, of these autoantibodies, the most important in detecting future type 1 diabetes are insulin autoantibodies (IAA), glutamic acid decarboxylase autoantibodies (GADA) and antibodies to insulinoma-associated autoantigen-2 (IA-2). The presence of IAA, GADA and IA-2 in addition to ICA greatly increases the risk of subsequent type 1 diabetes compared with the presence of ICA alone.

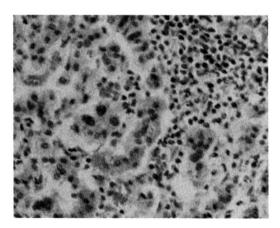

Figure 3.3 Type 1 diabetes results from a progressive loss of β cells as a consequence of chronic inflammation and destruction of the islets (insulitis), as shown in this histological section from a newly diagnosed patient.

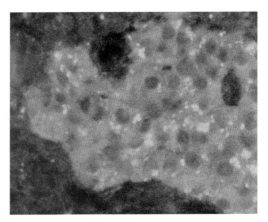

Figure 3.4 Islet cell antibodies in patients with type 1 diabetes can be detected with indirect immunofluorescence.

Immune destruction of β cells

Much of our understanding of the mechanism of β cell destruction has come from studies not in humans but in the non-obese diabetic (NOD) mouse and biobreeding (BB) rat, with the former now being the favored model of type 1 diabetes. Insulitis is associated with the presence of CD4+ and CD8+ T cells and macrophages, suggesting that these cells play an important role in the destruction of β cells. We know that the destructive process is very specific to β cells, with α cells being left intact.

In a commonly proposed model, a virus, dietary constituent or other unidentified agent initiates an abnormal immune response to pancreatic tissue. An aberrant expression of MHC class II antigens is generated. In response to this, T cells are activated and divide into two T helper subsets, termed Th1 and Th2. Th1 cells produce pro-inflammatory cytokines such as interleukin (IL)-2, interferon γ and tumor necrosis factor β. Th2 cells secrete IL-4, IL-5, IL-6 and IL-10. Such cytokines have been shown to exert toxic effects on the β cell and to inhibit insulin secretion. Th2 cells are responsible for B cell helper function, resulting in the production of the aforementioned antibodies directed against both the cytoplasmic components of islet cells and islet cell constituents. Experimental manipulation to prevent T cell responses in animal studies can also prevent the emergence of diabetes. 23

Some individuals may develop the autoimmune markers of type 1 diabetes but not go on to develop the disease; persistence of ICA, however, is associated with progressive β cell destruction and the emergence of clinical type 1 diabetes.

Loss of β cell mass

The autoimmune process in type 1 diabetes is associated with a decline in β cell mass. When this is sufficiently pronounced, insulin secretion becomes deficient, with a concomitant fall in C-peptide levels, leading eventually to symptomatic hyperglycemia (C-peptide is co-secreted with insulin). Once β cell destruction is advanced, C-peptide levels become undetectable although, as mentioned previously, C-peptide levels may be detectable in some patients for several months after the clinical diagnosis of type 1 diabetes. Autoantibody levels decline and, in most cases, the autoantibodies eventually disappear from the serum.

Hyperglycemia produces the classic symptoms with which people with type 1 diabetes present. Patients usually consult their doctor with osmotic symptoms of intense thirst, polydipsia and polyuria and complain of unintentional weight loss. Blurring of vision is very common at the time of diagnosis and is caused by osmotic effects on the lens of the eye. Rarely, and sadly, cases still present in diabetic ketoacidosis because the diagnosis of acute-onset type 1 diabetes has not been considered.

Key points – type 1 diabetes mellitus

- Type 1 diabetes results from an absolute deficiency of insulin.
- Osmotic symptoms at onset include thirst, polydipsia and polyuria.
- Environmental factors that cause the condition are unknown, but possibly include viral infection.
- Multiple inherited genetic factors influence both disease susceptibility and resistance.
- Autoimmune processes lead to β cell destruction and a decline in β cell mass.

Key references

Atkinson M. Type 1 diabetes: immunology. In: Wass JAH, Shalet SM, eds. Oxford *Textbook of Endocrinology and Diabetes*. Oxford: Oxford University Press, 2002:1659–69.

Atkinson MA, Eisenbarth GS. Type 1 diabetes: new perspective on disease pathogenesis and treatment. *Lancet* 2001;358:221–9.

Bain SC, Kelly MA, Mijovic CH, Barnett AH. Genetic factors in the pathogenesis of type 1 diabetes mellitus. In: Pickup J, Williams G, eds. *Textbook of Diabetes*, 3rd edn. Oxford: Blackwell Scientific Publications, 2003:15.1–14.

Foulis AK, Liddle CN, Farquharson MA et al. The histopathology of the pancreas in type 1 (insulin-dependent) diabetes mellitus: a 25-year review of deaths in patients under 20 years of age in the United Kingdom. *Diabetologia* 1986;29:267–74.

Pociot F, McDermott MF. Genetics of type 1 diabetes mellitus. *Genes Immun* 2002;3:235–49.

Yeung WC, Rawlinson WD, Craig ME. Enterovirus infection and type 1 diabetes mellitus: systematic review and meta-analysis of observational molecular studies. *BMJ* 2011;342:d35.

4   Type 2 diabetes mellitus

Type 2 diabetes occurs when insulin secretion is insufficient to meet insulin demand, resulting in hyperglycemia. The precedent pathophysiological events are characterized by varying degrees of metabolic derangement, which often differ in degrees between individuals. The keys are insulin resistance in muscle (thereby increasing insulin demand), insulin resistance in liver (thereby increasing hepatic gluconeogenesis) and eventual β cell failure with relative insulin deficiency (that is, unable to meet insulin demand). While there is relative insulin deficiency in type 2 diabetes, it is rarely absolute deficiency as in type 1 diabetes, thus ketoacidosis does not occur with hyperglycemia. The symptoms of type 2 diabetes are outlined in Table 4.1.

Type 2 diabetes is often considered a lifestyle disease. This is a misunderstanding, as type 2 diabetes has a strong genetic background, stronger in fact than that for type 1 diabetes. In monozygotic twins, there is a 95% concordance for type 2 diabetes; in contrast, the concordance for type 1 diabetes is 30–50%. The genetic predisposition

TABLE 4.1

Symptoms of type 2 diabetes mellitus

- Fatigue
- Polyuria
- Polydipsia
- Weight gain or weight loss
- Blurred vision
- Recurrent skin infections
  - fungal infections in skin creases
  - vulval or vaginal fungal infections
  - balanitis

for type 2 diabetes is, however, brought out very strongly by the environmental factors of a sedentary lifestyle, consumption of energy-dense foods and overweight or obesity.

Type 2 diabetes mellitus represents hyperglycemia, the end stage of β cell dysfunction, with numerous pathways to reach this endpoint. This has become evident as different genes have been found in different populations. Further, there are many different clinical phenotypes of the condition, varying from slim antibody-negative individuals who demonstrate the need for early insulin replacement, through to obese individuals whose hyperglycemia resolves with modest weight loss and minimal medication. There are often varying degrees of dyslipidemia and associated endocrine diseases such as polycystic ovary syndrome.

Genetics

Interestingly, most of the genes identified for type 2 diabetes concern the β cell. This indicates that the genetic predisposition for type 2 diabetes lies in a defect affecting insulin secretory capacity or the long-term ability to continue increased insulin secretion in the face of high demand or, perhaps, programming for long-term failure.

Mutational forms of type 2 diabetes explain only a small proportion of cases, fewer than 2%. These include the various forms of maturity onset diabetes of youth (MODY), which are covered in chapter 5. The mutations in certain genes *causing* monogenic forms of diabetes are listed in Table 4.2. In contrast, a number of different genetic polymorphisms have been described in different populations that explain *susceptibility* to the commoner forms of type 2 diabetes. These are also listed in Table 4.2.

Environmental

Environmental factors play a major role in increasing diabetes risk. These include a sedentary lifestyle, consumption of energy-dense foods and drinks (high carbohydrate and/or high fat) and obesity. Modifying these environmental factors is the focus of international public health efforts to curb the increasing global prevalence of type 2 diabetes and is the cornerstone of treatment and/or prevention of type 2 diabetes.

TABLE 4.2

Genetic mutations and genetic polymorphisms in type 2 diabetes mellitus

Single genes* (name [symbol])	Genetic polymorphisms associated with diabetes† (name [symbol])
• HNF1 homeobox A (*HNF1A*)	• Transcription factor 7-like 2 (T-cell specific, HMG-box) (*TCF7L2*)
• Hepatocyte nuclear factor 4, α (*HNF4A*)	• Peroxisome proliferator-activated receptor γ (*PPARG*)
• Glucokinase (hexokinase 4) (*GCK*)	• Calpain 10 (*CAPN10*)
	• Fat mass and obesity associated (*FTO*)

For more information, see www.ncbi.nlm.nih.gov/gene
*Mutations here cause diabetes.
†Not an exhaustive list.

The effectiveness of this approach is best demonstrated by the Diabetes Prevention Program, in which increased physical activity and modest weight reduction reduced the conversion of impaired glucose tolerance to type 2 diabetes by over 50% at 3 years.

Obesity has the strongest impact on promoting all forms of diabetes, including those without a clear genetic susceptibility.

Ethnic origin. In certain ethnic groups, loss of traditional lifestyles and adoption of a western diet have had catastrophic effects on prevalence rates, with the majority of adults now affected by type 2 diabetes. Ethnic groups including indigenous Australians, Nauruans (Pacific) and Pima Indians (USA) appear particularly susceptible. Adoption of a western lifestyle has also increased the susceptibility to type 2 diabetes among Hispanic Americans and populations in Southern and South East Asia, the Middle East and the Pacific Islands.

Pathogenesis

Insulin resistance is considered a central metabolic feature of many cases of type 2 diabetes. While it is often present in obesity-associated diabetes, it is not universal. In fact, insulin resistance is not present in many people with type 2 diabetes, particularly leaner individuals.

Insulin resistance accompanies abdominal obesity and is present in atherothrombotic cardiovascular disease. It accompanies dyslipidemia characterized by hypertriglyceridemia and low-HDL cholesterol, which is often found in type 2 diabetes, abdominal obesity and metabolic syndrome. Insulin resistance is considered the link that explains the clustering of abdominal obesity, type 2 diabetes, heart disease, hypertension and dyslipidemia.

Insulin resistance refers to the reduced ability of circulating insulin to result in cellular glucose uptake. Glucose serves as the major energy substrate for many tissues including muscle and the brain. Insulin acts by stimulating its receptor on the cell surface (Figure 4.1). This sets up a cascade of phosphorylation steps of subcellular enzymes that are controlled by key regulators. The eventual result is the movement of a glucose transporter, glucose transporter 4 (GLUT4), from the cell cytosol to the cell surface, and this permits glucose uptake into the cell (Figure 4.1). Within this complex pathway, there are many points at which signaling may be perturbed. Overall, such perturbation results in a reduced glucose-uptake response to insulin (insulin resistance).

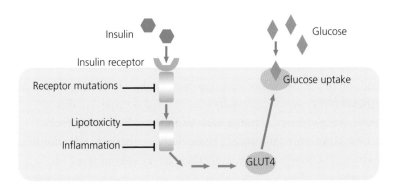

Figure 4.1 Cellular insulin-mediated glucose uptake and insulin resistance. Insulin receptor mutations, high intracellular lipid concentrations and inflammation block post-insulin receptor signaling that results in glucose uptake.

The body attempts to override this by producing more insulin (hyperinsulinemia). When the pancreatic β cells can no longer produce sufficient insulin to overcome insulin resistance, blood glucose levels start to rise.

Insulin resistance may occur at many points in the insulin signaling cascade. Rarely, genetic mutations within the insulin receptor or its substrate can result in insulin resistance. More frequently, increased circulating fatty acids (from nutrient excess or obesity) can interfere with insulin signaling through a mechanism termed lipotoxicity.

In addition, low-grade systemic inflammation is often found in obesity; disturbed adipose tissue secretion of molecules called adipokines (such as adiponectin, tumor necrosis factor α [TNFα], interleukin-6) can contribute to this. Adipokines can interfere with insulin action through a number of specific pathways involving intracellular inflammation signal transduction pathways that link in to insulin signaling pathways. These disturbances in inflammation add to the metabolic disturbances in the regulation of insulin signaling and contribute to insulin resistance.

Insulin resistance is also found in the liver. With failing insulin secretion, there is insufficient insulin to suppress hepatic gluconeogenesis, particularly overnight. This results in a rising fasting glucose: as the insulin secretory capacity diminishes, fasting glucose rises further (Figure 4.2). Insulin secretion is further hindered by rising glucose levels which directly damage β cells through a mechanism called glucotoxicity.

Lipotoxicity

Lipotoxicity in type 2 diabetes is found in the muscle cells, where glucose is the major substrate. However, it has also been reported in the pancreas, where the effects of excess lipid can contribute to damage to insulin-secreting β cells. Thus, in the situation of nutrient excess and obesity, where there are excess amounts of circulating fatty acids, lipotoxicity can increase insulin resistance (and the demand for insulin) *and* diminish the ability to respond by worsening β cell impairment (see Figure 4.2).

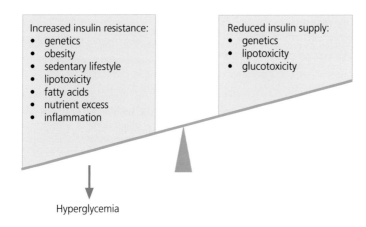

Hyperglycemia

Figure 4.2 Contributors to insulin demand–supply mismatch and hyperglycemia in type 2 diabetes.

Key points – type 2 diabetes mellitus

- Type 2 diabetes results from a relative deficiency of insulin, often in the context of insulin resistance.
- Nutrient excess and obesity contribute to insulin resistance, through mechanisms that include cell signaling defects, lipotoxicity and inflammation.
- As the pancreatic secretion of insulin starts to fail, glucose levels progressively rise due to dysregulation of hepatic gluconeogenesis.
- Multiple genetic factors predispose to type 2 diabetes; environmental factors such as obesity and a sedentary lifestyle accelerate its onset.

Key references

Crandall JP, Knowler WC, Kahn SE et al. The prevention of type 2 diabetes. *Nat Clin Pract Endocrinol Metab* 2008;4:382–93.

Guillausseau PJ, Meas T, Virally M et al. Abnormalities in insulin secretion in type 2 diabetes mellitus. *Diabetes Metab* 2008;34(suppl 2): S43–8.

Knowler WC, Barrett-Connor E, Fowler SE et al. Reduction in the incidence of type 2 diabetes with lifestyle intervention or metformin. *N Engl J Med* 2002;346:393–403.

Kraegen EW, Cooney GJ. Free fatty acids and skeletal muscle insulin resistance. *Curr Opin Lipidol* 2008;19:235–41.

Murphy R, Ellard S, Hattersley AT. Clinical implications of a molecular genetic classification of monogenic beta-cell diabetes. *Nat Clin Pract Endocrinol Metab* 2008;4:200–13.

Less common forms of diabetes mellitus may present with symptoms similar to those of type 1 or type 2 diabetes, but can have a number of diverse causes (Table 5.1).

Monogenic forms of diabetes mellitus

Monogenic forms of diabetes account for 1–2% of diabetes. These forms of diabetes, which result from mutations affecting β cell function, are commonly referred to as maturity onset diabetes of youth (MODY). It is important to consider these forms of diabetes, as their treatment requirements can differ and they can be misclassified as type 1 or 2 diabetes.

MODY is generally characterized by the onset of hyperglycemia at an early age (under 25 years) without ketoacidosis. The family history is usually positive for diabetes in two to three generations, which should raise the suspicion. Other suggestive features include the absence of autoantigens such as glutamic acid decarboxylase (GAD) or islet cell antibodies and detectable C-peptide. The lack of signs suggestive of insulin resistance – obesity, acanthosis nigricans and polycystic ovary syndrome – should also raise suspicion. MODY can be distinguished into types detected at birth and types detected later in life.

Neonatal hyperglycemia. Individuals diagnosed before the age of 6 months are more likely to have monogenic diabetes than autoimmune β cell destruction (type 1 diabetes). Neonatal hyperglycemia is mostly due to mutations in the ATP-sensitive potassium channel (Kir6.2 and SUR1 subunits). This form of monogenic diabetes is best treated with oral sulfonylurea medication rather than insulin. Thus, making an accurate diagnosis in these circumstances affects clinical treatment. The majority of these cases occur as spontaneous mutations, and there is usually no family history.

TABLE 5.1

Classification of other causes of diabetes mellitus

Gestational diabetes mellitus*

Genetic defects

β cell function

- HNF1A (chr. 12) (MODY3)
- Glucokinase (chr. 7) (MODY2)
- HNF4A (chr. 20) (MODY1)
- Insulin promoter factor-1 (chr. 13) (MODY4) and others

Insulin action

- Type A insulin resistance
- Leprechaunism
- Lipoatrophic diabetes
- Others

Pancreatic disease

- Pancreatitis
- Cystic fibrosis
- Hemochromatosis
- Pancreatic carcinoma

Drug-induced

- Glucocorticoids
- Combined antiretroviral therapy for HIV
- Nicotinic acid
- Pentamidine
- Diazoxide
- Thyroxine and others

Endocrinopathies

- Acromegaly
- Cushing's syndrome
- Pheochromocytoma
- Hyperthyroidism
- Glucagonoma
- Somatostatinoma

Infections

- Congenital rubella
- Cytomegalovirus

Transplantation-associated diabetes

Genetic syndromes associated with diabetes

- Down's syndrome
- Klinefelter's syndrome
- Turner's syndrome
- Wolfram's syndrome
- Friedrich's ataxia
- Prader–Willi syndrome

*Gestational diabetes mellitus is discussed in detail in chapter 12.
Chr, chromosome.
American Diabetes Association 2011.

Familial fasting hyperglycemia. Mutations in the glucokinase gene results in familial mild fasting hyperglycemia (MODY2). This condition can be present from birth and asymptomatic and it does not require any specific treatment. It is often detected when children or adolescents have investigations for other reasons. Microvascular complications are rare. Treatment is generally not required.

Hepatic nuclear factor mutations. Mutations in the genes encoding hepatic nuclear factors (HNFs), which are transcription factors, result in MODY1 (*HNF4A*), MODY3 (*HNF1A*) or MODY5 (*HNF1B*). There is often a strong family history of diabetes and the onset of hyperglycemia before the age of 25 years. Genetic analysis for diagnosis is useful for these patients as the diagnosis can alter clinical management.

HNF1A mutations (or MODY3) produce diabetes in adolescence or early adulthood. Glycosuria is present early on, even before the development of hyperglycemia. Fasting glucose levels can be normal early on and postprandial hyperglycemia can be exaggerated. With progressive β cell failure, fasting hyperglycemia develops. Microvascular complications in this form of MODY are predicted by glycemic control, just as for type 1 and type 2 diabetes. Interestingly, patients with this mutation appear to be more susceptible to ischemic heart disease, despite having the elevated HDL cholesterol that characterizes the condition.

HNF1B (or MODY5) is the most common form of monogenic diabetes due to transcription factor mutation. Estimates suggest it accounts for 1% of all diabetes. It is particularly responsive to sulfonylurea therapy, even at very low doses, which is why accurate diagnosis is necessary. It also has a very high penetrance, again necessitating accurate diagnosis and making genetic counseling important.

HNF4A (or MODY1) mutations produce diabetes that appears very similar to that arising from mutations in *HNF1A*, with the distinction of a different lipid pattern. Reduced levels of lipoprotein A1, lipoprotein A2 and HDL cholesterol are found. Again, diagnosis assists in clinical management as this form of diabetes responds to low-dose sulfonylurea therapy.

35

Diabetes mellitus associated with other endocrine diseases

Diabetes can also occur in the context of other underlying endocrine diseases, such as Cushing's syndrome, acromegaly, thyrotoxicosis and pheochromocytoma. Clinical features of these conditions should be sought at diagnosis of diabetes, with biochemical confirmation. Treatment of the underlying condition usually results in amelioration of the hyperglycemia.

Pancreatic disease

Conditions affecting the integrity of the pancreas can damage β cells and result in hyperglycemia. These conditions include cystic fibrosis, hemochromatosis and pancreatic carcinoma. A patient may already have the diagnosis, as in the case of cystic fibrosis, or a condition such as hemochromatosis can be considered at diagnosis, particularly if there are features of skin pigmentation, hepatomegaly and a history of fatigue and degenerative joint disease. Pancreatic carcinoma should be considered in the older individual who also has weight loss.

Drug-induced diabetes mellitus

Hyperglycemia can result from a number of drugs that affect either insulin secretion or insulin action.

Glucocorticoids reduce insulin action, even at low doses. Glucocorticoids can unmask an underlying susceptibility to type 2 diabetes, but can also induce hyperglycemia if used at high enough doses. Glucocorticoid-induced hyperglycemia can have a characteristic pattern of normal (or even low) fasting glucose levels and pronounced hyperglycemia by mid-afternoon (in those patients receiving morning doses). It usually ameliorates in the days or weeks after glucocorticoid cessation.

Anti-HIV drugs also increase insulin resistance. They include the protease inhibitors and nucleoside reverse transcriptase inhibitors. Studies indicate that within each of these drug classes, different drugs are more likely to worsen insulin resistance. HIV infection treated with combined antiretroviral therapy (cART) is associated with an increased risk of diabetes, with some studies indicating a fourfold increase.

Pentamidine, a drug used to treat pneumocystis infection in AIDS, is a β cell toxin that has also been associated with inducing ketosis-prone diabetes that requires ongoing insulin therapy.

Transplantation-associated diabetes mellitus

Solid organ transplantation is also associated with diabetes mellitus and can be attributed to glucocorticoid use; however, some of the immunosuppressants used in transplantation have also been implicated. Recipients of renal and cardiac transplantation appear particularly susceptible. Lung recipients (particularly those with underlying cystic fibrosis) are also at higher risk because of underlying damage to the exocrine pancreas.

Others

A number of genetic syndromes that can be associated with diabetes mellitus and other causes, such as infections, are listed in Table 5.1.

Key points – other types of diabetes mellitus

- Onset of hyperglycemia without ketoacidosis in non-obese individuals under 25 years of age is suggestive of MODY. A positive family history of diabetes in two to three generations should raise this suspicion.
- Conditions such as cystic fibrosis, hemochromatosis and pancreatic carcinoma can cause hyperglycemia.
- Glucocorticoids can unmask a susceptibility to type 2 diabetes or cause hyperglycemia at high doses. Anti-HIV drugs increase insulin resistance. Pentamidine can cause ketosis-prone diabetes.
- Renal, cardiac and lung transplantation increases the risk of diabetes.

Key references

American Diabetes Association. Standards of care. Causes and diagnosis of diabetes mellitus. *Diabetes Care* 2011;34(suppl 1): S12–15.

Vaxillaire M, Froguel P. Monogenic diabetes in the young, pharmacogenetics and relevance to multifactorial forms of type 2 diabetes. *Endocr Rev* 2008;29: 254–64.

A diagnosis of type 1 diabetes changes the lives of affected patients for ever. Many face the prospect of injecting themselves with insulin for the rest of their lives with considerable dread. In time, however, virtually all patients accommodate to the prospect of daily self-injection with a degree of fortitude; indeed, it is the minority of patients who live their lives in complete resentment of their condition.

Insulin treatment for type 1 diabetes aims to lower glucose levels in the blood to as near to the normal (non-diabetic) range as possible (Figure 6.1) without causing significant hypoglycemia. The objectives of this strategy are to:

- maintain body weight
- avoid hyperglycemic symptoms
- delay or prevent the onset of complications of diabetes
- prevent patients from developing diabetic ketoacidosis.

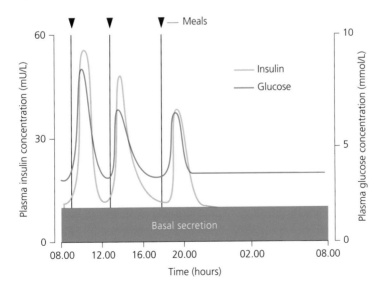

Figure 6.1 Physiological plasma insulin and glucose profiles in the fed and fasted states.

Evidence to support such a strategy emerged in 1993 following the publication of the landmark Diabetes Control and Complications Trial (DCCT) in the USA, which established beyond reasonable doubt that intensive insulin therapy delays the onset and slows the progression of specific diabetic microvascular complications.

In practice, achieving normal blood glucose levels is not possible even with multiple-injection or insulin pump therapy, and achieving near-normal blood glucose values in a 24-hour period poses a formidable challenge to all but a small minority of patients. In this context, the role of the diabetes team is to help patients approach or reach this goal while providing professional and holistic support and guidance along the way.

Insulin regimens

Animal-derived insulins (both porcine and bovine) are used by a diminishing minority of patients with a long duration of diabetes. Most patients with type 1 diabetes are treated with a variety of human insulin preparations or, increasingly, recombinant insulin analogs. Patients using animal insulins sometimes maintain that using human insulin produced either by enzymatic modification or recombinant-DNA technology is associated with lack of awareness of hypoglycemia. However, this phenomenon has not been reported in the USA and the hypothesis has largely been patient driven. There is no scientific evidence to support this contention, though current practice is to support patients who choose to continue using animal insulin as no material harm will ensue. Only a few manufacturers continue to produce insulin derived from animals. No major world insulin producer continues to do so.

Rapidly acting insulins such as the insulin analog insulin lispro (Humalog) have an onset of action of 5–10 minutes and a duration of action of 3–4 hours. Intermediate-acting insulins such as the isophane insulins act within 30–60 minutes and continue to act for 9–12 hours. Insulin glargine (Lantus), a more truly basal insulin, has an onset of action after 5 hours and will act for more than 24 hours in most cases, while insulin detemir (Levemir) acts after 60 minutes and lasts for

24 hours. The biphasic insulin analogs have an onset of action of 10–20 minutes and a duration of up to 24 hours. Rapidly acting insulin analogs can be injected just as the meal is eaten, but it is preferable to inject the other insulins 30–40 minutes before eating in order to match the absorption of insulin into the bloodstream with the rise in blood glucose levels on eating. Table 6.1 lists some common insulin preparations.

Delivery methods and injection sites. Insulin is available in vials from which the insulin is drawn up and injected subcutaneously using lightweight sterilized disposable insulin syringes and matched needles (Figure 6.2). In many countries, the majority of patients use reusable insulin pen injectors fitted with cartridges (Figure 6.3) or convenient preloaded pens (Figure 6.4). The usual sites recommended for insulin injection are illustrated in Figure 6.5. It is preferable for short-acting insulins to be injected into the abdomen and for longer-acting insulins to be injected into the thigh area.

Basal–bolus regimens (multiple dose injection) of insulin administration were developed in response to the perceived rigidity and lack of flexibility of older regimens incorporating isophane insulins or fixed mixtures, with their inherent predisposition to hypoglycemia, especially mid-morning and mid-afternoon.

Basal–bolus refers to a multiple-dose regimen whereby insulin with a rapid but short duration of action is injected subcutaneously with breakfast, lunch and the evening meal (bolus insulin) and a long-acting (basal) insulin is injected usually, but not exclusively, before bed. In addition to the theoretical advantage in terms of blood glucose control, such regimens were further fostered by significant developments in insulin pen delivery devices and the development of modern short- and long-acting insulin analogs. An example of such a regimen would be insulin aspart (NovoRapid) or insulin lispro injected with meals, and insulin detemir or insulin glargine injected before bed. Sometimes the long-acting insulin is injected twice daily, 12 hours apart, to achieve better basal blood glucose control.

TABLE 6.1

Commonly used insulin preparations for subcutaneous use

Short-acting insulins

Human monocomponent insulins
- (Novolin R/Actrapid)
- (Humulin R/Humulin S)
- (Insuman Rapid [not available in USA])

Recombinant human insulin analogs
- Insulin aspart (NovoLog/NovoRapid)
- Insulin lispro (Humalog)
- Insulin glulisine (Apidra)

Intermediate- and long-acting insulins

Human monocomponent insulins
- Isophane insulin (Novolin N/Insulatard; Humulin N/Humulin I; Insuman Basal [not in USA])

Recombinant human insulins
- Insulin detemir (Levemir)
- Insulin glargine (Lantus)

Biphasic insulins

- (Novolin 70/30)
- (Humulin 70/30/Humulin M3)
- (Insuman Comb 50 [not in USA])
- (NovoLog Mix 70/30/NovoMix 30)
- (Humalog Mix75/25/Humalog Mix25)

Proprietary names in brackets (USA/UK).

Basal–bolus regimens have, in recent years, become the most widely used method of insulin administration for the treatment of type 1 diabetes, particularly by younger patients with busy, active and, at times, irregular lives. The flexibility of such regimens allows patients

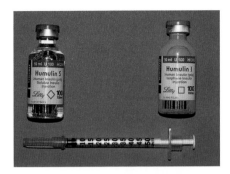

Figure 6.2 Vials of insulin with a lightweight plastic disposable syringe.*

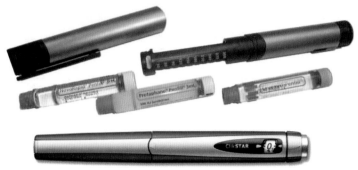

Figure 6.3 Reusable insulin pens are fitted with compact cartridges, which hold 150 or 300 units of insulin. The pens can be used for several years, and the cartridges generally take up less fridge space than preloaded pens.*

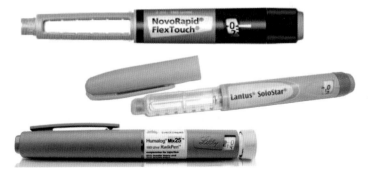

Figure 6.4 Disposable insulin pens are preloaded with insulin (most hold 300 units) and thrown away when empty. They are generally more convenient than reusable pens, and some enable half-unit adjustment of dose, which can be useful in children.*

*Photographs reproduced courtesy of Eli Lilly, NovoNordisk and Sanofi, UK.   43

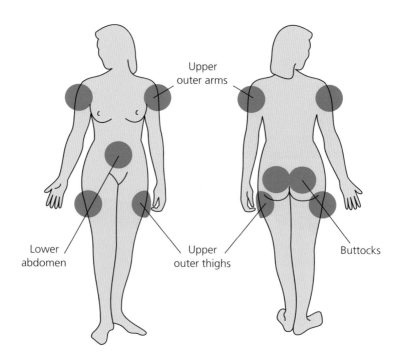

Figure 6.5 Subcutaneous insulin injection sites.

to eat at different times of the day without compromising glycemic control: the bolus insulin is injected when the patient eats to counter the expected post-meal glucose excursion, while glucose levels in the fasted state are kept under control by the long-acting basal insulin.

The availability of the basal insulins glargine and detemir has afforded a significant advance in the treatment of type 1 diabetes. These insulins have a more reproducible biological effect in daily use than isophane insulin preparations (such as Novolin N [also known as Insulatard] and Humulin N [also known as Humulin I]), which some patients still use as basal insulin, and this advantage has been associated with a lower incidence of nocturnal hypoglycemia. Furthermore, the use of very quick-acting insulin analogs has lessened the risk of delayed hypoglycemia in, for example, the late morning or afternoon.

Twice-daily fixed-mixture regimens comprise injections of a biphasic insulin, such as biphasic insulin lispro (25% insulin lispro, 75% insulin lispro protamine [Humalog Mix25]) or biphasic insulin aspart (30% insulin aspart, 70% insulin aspart protamine [NovoMix 30]) at breakfast and at the evening meal. Clearly this insulin regimen has the advantage of simplicity and hence it has been popular with children and the elderly. However, the lack of flexibility of this regimen means it does not lend itself well to young active patients, particularly those with an irregular lifestyle where the basal–bolus regimen confers considerable advantage.

In general, two-thirds of the total daily insulin dose is administered in the morning and one-third in the evening, though the ratio is subject to change according to the pattern of self-monitored blood glucose results. Such monitoring may also demonstrate the desirability of changing the ratio of short-acting to intermediate-acting insulins, and other preparations are available to allow this to be achieved. These include other biphasic insulins such as biphasic insulin lispro (50% insulin lispro, 50% insulin lispro protamine [Humalog Mix50]).

Less commonly, patients inject different insulins at different doses at breakfast and dinner, either separately or mixed in the same syringe (e.g. twice-daily doses of soluble insulin [Novolin R, also known as Actrapid] and isophane insulin [Novolin N, also known as Insulatard]). The drawback of twice-daily insulin regimens, either free or in a fixed mixture, is that their inherent inflexibility makes it necessary to eat at fixed times of the day, including mid-morning and mid-afternoon snacks, in order to avoid hypoglycemia. Such regimens may also be associated with a risk of nocturnal hypoglycemia as the peak effect of the intermediate insulin occurs between midnight and 03:00 hours, when the need for insulin is lowest. Failure of these regimens to produce adequate glycemic control without disabling hypoglycemia usually necessitates a switch to a basal–bolus regimen.

Other insulin combinations include three daily injections of fixed mixtures or a fixed mixture at breakfast, a short-acting insulin at dinner and a longer-acting insulin before bed, but such regimens are very much the province of specialized diabetes teams.

Developments

Novel insulin analogs will continue to be developed to help 'fine tune' the treatment by subcutaneous insulin injections. One such analog is insulin degludec, which has an ultra-long-acting profile attributable to the formation of soluble multihexamers at the injection site. A 16-week open-label trial comparing the efficacy of insulin degludec injected once daily or three times a week with that of insulin glargine injected once daily showed no difference in terms of achieved glycated hemoglobin HbA_{1c}, but with fewer participants experiencing hypoglycemia in the insulin degludec once-daily group than in the other groups. How such insulins will ultimately be used in clinical practice remains to be determined.

Insulin pumps

Insulin pumps have long been available to treat type 1 diabetes. They attempt to emulate physiological insulin levels by delivering a continuous subcutaneous insulin infusion (CSII) augmented by meal-related boluses of insulin.

The individual wears a small portable battery-driven pump (Figure 6.6) with a reservoir of rapidly acting insulin. Insulin is pumped down a delivery cannula, at the end of which is attached a fine-gauge 'butterfly' needle device that is inserted subcutaneously into the anterior abdominal wall. This needs to be re-sited every 1–2 days to avoid local inflammation. The pump delivers a predetermined basal insulin infusion (the rate of which can be varied during the 24-hour period), supplemented at meal times by a patient-activated bolus of short-acting insulin to provide a prandial boost. The basal rate of infusion and the bolus doses administered as prandial boosts are determined after a comprehensive education program delivered by the hospital-based insulin pump team. Such teams need to be available to offer telephone advice on a 24-hour basis in case of problems. Systems such as the Medtronic MiniMed Paradigm Real-Time insulin pump system (see Figure 6.6) have been developed to integrate the insulin delivered through the pump with continuous real-time glucose monitoring.

Studies consistently demonstrate that CSII treatment of type 1 diabetes produces a slight but significant improvement in blood

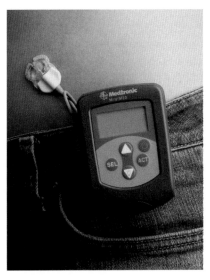

Figure 6.6 A patient fitted with the Medtronic MiniMed Paradigm Real-Time insulin pump system, which integrates insulin delivery through a pump with real-time continuous glucose monitoring. Reproduced courtesy of Medtronic, UK.

glucose control compared with basal–bolus regimens using pen devices. CSII is generally associated with lower rates of hypoglycemic episodes. It may be particularly suitable for patients experiencing recurrent troublesome hypoglycemia with multiple-injection regimens.

Disadvantages include the necessity to set up a special insulin pump service and the expense of funding the pumps and associated consumables. System malfunction can also arise, leading to the rapid development of diabetic ketoacidosis owing to the short half-life of insulin once it has entered the circulation. In recent years, however, experienced pump centers have reported a significant decrease in the rates of ketoacidosis in their patients, to the extent that it is no longer such an important problem. In some healthcare systems, diabetic patients have to satisfy certain criteria before pump therapy will be sanctioned for funding. Skin complications are encountered occasionally.

Patients who may gain considerable benefits from CSII include those with poor control on conventional therapy despite adequate education and support from the diabetes team, patients with erratic and unstable blood glucose control and those with unpredictable and recurrent hypoglycemia that has not been eradicated with the usual conventional approaches. CSII therapy is also used successfully by

47

pregnant diabetic women who find difficulty achieving recommended blood glucose targets with conventional subcutaneous insulin regimens. It may be particularly beneficial if hypoglycemia has been intractable with conventional insulin therapy during the pregnancy.

Insulin pump therapy is recommended as a treatment for children under 12 years of age when multiple injection treatment is considered impractical or inappropriate.

Patient choice is another valid reason for pump treatment, but this may pose a problem in some countries where funding may not be available on these grounds. CSII usage varies greatly between countries in the developed world, with particularly high usage rates in the USA and certain European countries. Many patients decline the choice of treating their diabetes with a pump for a variety of reasons. One frequently cited reason is that the physical presence of the pump, although small, is a constant reminder of the diabetic condition. It is likely that pump usage will increase, particularly in current low-usage countries such as the UK (about 4% of patients). It is estimated that 10–15% of patients would fulfill the criteria for pump therapy, although without conditions patient choice might drive this figure much higher.

Insulin allergy

Generalized allergy to insulin is rare but local allergic reactions may occur at the site of the injection causing local erythema, burning, pruritus, pain and induration. Such reactions usually respond to switching to a different insulin preparation. More common is the development of localized fat atrophy or hypertrophy at insulin injection sites, usually when the patient repeatedly uses the same site for injection. Patients need to be advised at the initiation of insulin treatment to rotate injection sites.

Needle phobia

Several devices are available on the market for those individuals who find the self-injection of insulin difficult. The Autoject 2, for example, automatically inserts the needle and contents of an insulin syringe into the skin without the patient having to see the needle. Insulin jet injectors are needle-free devices that project a fine spray of insulin through the skin at high pressure, although experience with such devices has not proven to be very satisfactory. The Insuflon Subcutaneous Injection Port is a soft flexible Teflon catheter that is inserted into the skin for periods of up to 5 days. Injections are administered through the silicone sealing membrane at the end of the device, thus avoiding the pain of injection. This device may be particularly helpful for use with young children.

Pancreatic transplantation

The first successful transplantation of a pancreas with simultaneous kidney transplantation was performed at the University of Minnesota in 1966. Now, about 1200 pancreas transplants are undertaken annually in the USA. Successful whole-pancreas transplantation has the ability to rid diabetic patients of the daily tedium of subcutaneous insulin injections and, where normal blood glucose levels are obtained, the need to make blood glucose measurements.

Pancreatic transplantation involves either a simultaneous pancreas–kidney (SPK) transplant or a pancreas transplant alone (PTA). The majority of pancreatic transplants are SPKs and, worldwide, many thousands of these procedures have been performed with considerable success that reflects improved surgical techniques and advances in immunosuppressive therapy. Figures quoted for actuarial survival of patients and functional pancreas grafts with complete independence from insulin for SPK recipients are 94% and 89%, respectively, at 1 year and 81% and 67% at 5 years. Some centers have been enthusiastic advocates of PTA, but the results for pancreas graft survival are lower than with SPK. SPK remains a very useful treatment strategy for those patients with end-stage kidney disease. As for other transplants, the shortage of donor organs remains a significant problem.

Islet cell transplantation

Islet cell transplantation, which has long been a proposed treatment strategy to replace lost β cell function, involves the transplantation of freshly prepared human islets (Figure 6.7) by embolization into the

49

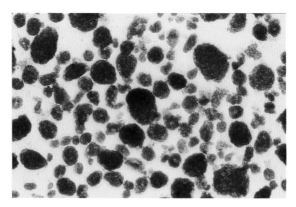

Figure 6.7 Freshly prepared islets, stained in red, ready to be transplanted. Reproduced courtesy of Professor Stephanie Amiel and Dr Guo Cai Huang, King's College Hospital, London, UK.

liver through a small catheter placed under fluoroscopic guidance into the main portal vein.

The success of this technique depends on the skillful preparation of human islets and the regimen of immunosuppression involved. A major advance in islet cell transplantation came in 2001 when a group in Edmonton, Canada, reported vastly superior results using a novel steroid-free immunosuppressive regimen consisting of pre- and post-transplant daclizumab (an anti-interleukin-2-receptor monoclonal antibody), maintenance sirolimus and low-dose tacrolimus. The Edmonton workers reported a 1-year rate of sustained insulin independence of 85%; at present, many centers throughout the world, including several in the UK, are attempting to emulate the success of this group.

As for whole-organ transplantation, the availability of donor pancreases will limit the usefulness and widespread application of this technique. Intriguingly, if very successful, islet cell transplantation could, in theory, reduce the need for SPK and PTA, while the prospect of improved treatment of diabetes may well obviate the need for both.

Self-monitoring of blood glucose

Patient self-monitoring of blood glucose is necessary to measure the effect of the administered doses of insulin on blood glucose levels. This is necessary to attempt to avoid hypoglycemia and to achieve blood glucose levels as near to the non-diabetic state as possible ('diabetic control'), or blood glucose targets mutually agreed by the patient and their physician.

Blood glucose meters measure the concentration of glucose by a variety of methods, but all require the collection of a very small quantity of capillary blood, usually from a fingertip. This is delivered on to a measuring strip that is then inserted into the meter for measurement. Blood glucose meters have become smaller, quicker and ever more sophisticated (an example is shown in Figure 6.8), but the technique of pricking a finger to produce a small sample of blood remains an unpleasant experience that is usually considered more painful than subcutaneous injection of insulin. Not surprisingly, this inhibits some patients from performing the requisite number of blood tests to manage their diabetic condition effectively. Although blood glucose meters achieve clinically acceptable standards of accuracy and precision under laboratory conditions, patients (and indeed doctors and nurses) may not replicate such standards, and this emphasizes the need for proper instruction in the technique of blood glucose measurement and regular assessment of quality control.

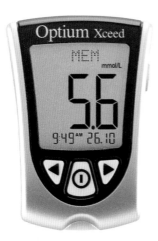

Figure 6.8 An example of a home glucose meter used for self-monitoring. Reproduced courtesy of Abbott Diabetes Care, UK.

Frequency and timing. Universal agreement as to how many blood glucose tests a person with insulin-treated diabetes should do to achieve good control is lacking. Suggestions include:

- two readings per day with variation of the timing of readings on alternate days
- four readings per day
- an intensive profile of four or more readings per day on selected days during the week.

Guidelines from a recent consensus conference suggest that patients taking multiple daily injections or using insulin pumps test three to four times daily. Patients using less frequent injections could test less often, as suggested above. Intercurrent illness, changes in insulin dose, a change in insulin regimen, preconception and pregnancy necessitate more frequent and intensive blood testing. Studies have shown an association with the number of blood tests performed and the glycated hemoglobin (HbA$_{1c}$) level: patients who tested more frequently had a lower HbA$_{1c}$ level. Occasionally, in some patients, blood testing can become excessive, obsessive and hence counterproductive.

Blood glucose measurements are taken immediately before meals, 2 hours after eating and before bed. Occasional testing during the night can be helpful to detect nocturnal hypoglycemia. Pregnant patients are often advised to check 1 hour after meals in some national guidelines. Patients use the results to determine whether insulin dose adjustment is necessary to reach predetermined targets (such as blood glucose values of 4–7 mmol/L [72–126 mg/dL] before the next meal) or to avoid hypoglycemia. Patients may also test at other times if they suspect they have symptoms of hypoglycemia. Although most patients develop the necessary skills to self-monitor blood glucose, some never adequately develop the skill of using the blood results to make appropriate changes to their insulin dosages. Intensive education courses may help patients to achieve such skills and all patients with type 1 diabetes should have access to such courses.

The future. Further tangible benefits of self-monitoring include allowing the patient to recognize the symptoms of hypoglycemia, the expected increase in blood glucose levels following the consumption of different foods and drinks and the blood glucose fall after various forms of physical exercise.

What patients with insulin-treated diabetes would like, however, is the ability to know their blood glucose concentration on a minute-by-minute basis. Many companies throughout the world are attempting to develop systems to allow this but, to date, no such system is available outside of the clinical research arena. Medtronic produce a system that allows continuous glucose monitoring; it measures interstitial glucose, which is in close equilibrium with plasma glucose. A sensor is implanted subcutaneously and is connected to a monitor/microprocessor device worn externally (Figure 6.9). The glucose data are downloaded on to a computer later and the observed patterns of glucose excursions are used to adjust insulin doses or regimens and to detect periods of unrecognized hypoglycemia (Figure 6.10). Surprising profiles of blood glucose are often found that could never have been anticipated from normal self-monitoring.

Testing for ketones

Patients are taught how to check for the presence of ketones in special situations such as when self-monitored blood glucose levels are very high and during concurrent illness. Ketone testing is also very useful

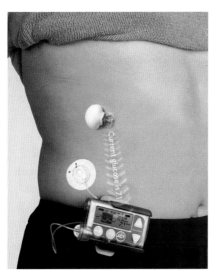

Figure 6.9 The MiniMed continuous-glucose-monitoring system. Reproduced courtesy of Medtronic, UK.

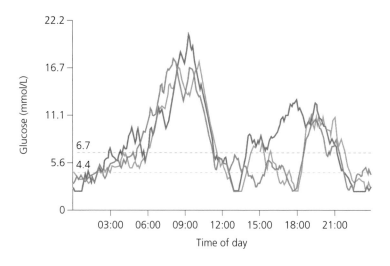

Figure 6.10 Downloaded 24-hour glucose profiles using the MiniMed continuous-glucose-monitoring system. Reproduced courtesy of Medtronic, UK.

in young children. Traditionally, urine was tested for ketones using proprietary strips but now the Optium Xceed meter has a facility that allows blood ketones to be quantified from a capillary sample. When moderate ketonemia is detected, advice from appropriately trained staff may be sufficient to help the person correct the ketosis and thus avoid hospital admission. The finding of high levels of ketones in the blood will warrant urgent admission to hospital to prevent the development of significant diabetic ketoacidosis.

HbA$_{1c}$

Further to the problems associated with self-monitoring of blood glucose outlined above, HbA$_{1c}$ measurement has become the gold standard for the assessment of diabetes control. Glycated (or glycosylated) hemoglobin refers to a series of minor hemoglobin components (HbA$_{1a}$, HbA$_{1b}$ and HbA$_{1c}$) formed by the adduction of glucose to normal adult hemoglobin.

Quantitatively, HbA$_{1c}$ is the most important of these minor components and hence it has become the component used to assess glycemic control. HbA_{1c} reflects the integrated blood glucose concentration over a period that approximates to the half-life of the red cell (i.e. 6–8 weeks), and thus HbA_{1c} measurement allows assessment of long-term diabetes control. The more glucose in the circulation, the greater the production of glycated hemoglobin.

Any medical condition that decreases red-cell survival (such as acute or chronic blood loss or hemolytic anemia) will tend to result in lower HbA_{1c} values, so results may need to be interpreted with caution. Similarly, spurious results may be obtained in patients with a hemoglobinopathy. For example, hemoglobin F, as is present in β-thalassemia, will be measured with HbA_{1c} in certain laboratory assays, giving rise to misleadingly high results. HbA_{1c} may also be an unreliable marker of glycemic control in the presence of renal failure. An alternative index of glycemic control in patients with blood loss, hemolytic anemia or hemoglobinopathy is measurement of serum fructosamine (glycated serum protein). Fructosamine is not affected by such conditions and reflects glycemia in the preceding 2–3 weeks, allowing an assessment of more rapid change in blood glucose levels.

HbA_{1c} results have traditionally been reported as a percentage of total hemoglobin. Following the development of an internationally recognized standard reference method, HbA_{1c} is now reported as millimoles of HbA_{1c} per mole of Hb, with an HbA_{1c} of 53 mmol/mol being the equivalent of a DCCT-aligned HbA_{1c} of 7% (DCCT is the Diabetes Control and Complications Trial).

Normal self-monitored blood glucose values in the face of an elevated HbA_{1c} usually imply a patient's falsification of their results, an inability to perform blood glucose tests properly, a fault in the blood glucose meter or a spurious HbA_{1c} result. HbA_{1c} should be measured every 4–6 months in patients with type 1 diabetes to make judgments about glycemic control and the need for modification of the insulin regimen.

Targets. The American Diabetes Association recommends that patients try to achieve an HbA_{1c} below 53 mmol/mol (7%). However, other professional bodies recommend different targets. The Joint British Societies advocate an HbA_{1c} target below 48 mmol/mol (6.5%) (with an audit standard of lower than 59 mmol/mol [7.5%]). The target of the International Diabetes Federation (Europe) is less than or equal to 48 mmol/mol (6.5%), while the National Institute for Health and Clinical Excellence (NICE), for England and Wales, specifies that the target HbA_{1c} should be in the range 48–59 mmol/mol (6.5–7.5%). Ideally, the HbA_{1c} should be lowered to the upper limit of the normal non-diabetic range, but in practice this is usually not achievable because of the associated risk of hypoglycemia.

Less stringent targets for HbA_{1c} may be appropriate for those of advanced age, those with significant comorbid conditions, children, patients with a history of severe hypoglycemia, patients with limited life expectancy and patients with longstanding diabetes and minimal or stable microvascular complications. In good clinical practice the patient and their physician should agree on a specified target HbA_{1c} based on a shared knowledge of the patient's circumstances.

The role of diabetes education

Properly evaluated methods of educating patients with type 1 diabetes in the principles of diabetes self-management are essential if individuals are to achieve HbA_{1c} targets without hypoglycemia. This was reinforced by the experience of participants in the DCCT.

Education is best delivered by a multidisciplinary team comprising dietitians, diabetes nurse educators and diabetologists. A paradigm for the education of patients with type 1 diabetes is the Dose Adjustment for Normal Eating (DAFNE) program pioneered in Düsseldorf, Germany. This evidence-based program is now being delivered with good results by accredited DAFNE training centers in many European countries. Most patients find the DAFNE course to be self-empowering, and attendance has been consistently shown to lead to an improved quality of life, greater freedom of choice with food and, at least in the short term, a fall in HbA_{1c} level.

Education methods should include open access, support, encouragement, motivational strategies and coping-oriented techniques. Psychosocial problems associated with type 1 diabetes, which are relatively common, may need to be specifically addressed.

Despite this, it must be recognized that many patients will only achieve suboptimal control of their diabetes while others will, even with a great deal of input from specialist teams, have chronically poor diabetes control.

Key points – treatment of type 1 diabetes mellitus

- Insulin treatment of type 1 diabetes attempts to keep plasma glucose levels as near normal as possible without causing hypoglycemia.
- Most young patients are treated with a basal–bolus regimen incorporating rapid-acting insulin analogs at mealtimes and a basal long-acting insulin analog.
- Twice-daily fixed-mixture regimens may be useful for children and the elderly.
- Pump therapy is a very effective and safe mode of treatment for some patients.
- Pancreatic and islet cell transplantation may be offered to highly selected type 1 patients.
- Insulin therapy confers the need to perform self-monitoring of blood glucose levels.
- Diabetes control is assessed by regular measurement of glycated hemoglobin (HbA_{1c}).
- Diabetes education programs help diabetic patients to manage their condition more effectively.

Key references

American Diabetes Association. Summary of Revisions for the 2008 Clinical Practice Recommendations. *Diabetes Care* 2008;31:S3–4.

Bergenstal RM, Gavin JR 3rd; Global Consensus Conference on Glucose Monitoring Panel. The role of self-monitoring of blood glucose in the care of people with diabetes: report of a global consensus conference. *Am J Med* 2005; 118(suppl 9A):1S–6S.

Bolli GB. Insulin treatment and its complications. In: Pickup J, Williams G, eds. *Textbook of Diabetes*, 3rd edn, Oxford: Blackwell Scientific Publications, 2003:43.1–43.20.

DAFNE study group. Training in flexible, intensive insulin management to enable dietary freedom in people with type 1 diabetes: dose adjustment for normal eating (DAFNE) randomized controlled trial. *BMJ* 2002;325: 746–8.

DeVries JH, Snoek FJ, Heine RJ. Persistent poor glycaemic control in adult type 1 diabetes. A closer look at the problem. *Diabetic Med* 2004;21:1263–8.

The Diabetes Control and Complications Trial Research Group. The effect of intensive treatment of diabetes on the development and progression of long-term complications in insulin-dependent diabetes mellitus. *N Engl J Med* 1993;329:977–86.

Karter AJ, Ackerson LM, Darbinian JA et al. Self-monitoring of blood glucose levels and glycemic control: the Northern California Kaiser Permanente Diabetes Registry. *Am J Med* 2001;111:1–9.

National Institute for Health and Clinical Excellence (NICE). Type 1 diabetes: diagnosis and management of type 1 diabetes in children, young people and adults. Clinical Guideline 15. Available from www.nice.org.uk/nicemedia/pdf/CG015NICE guidelines, last accessed 22 November 2011.

Robertson PR. Islet cell transplantation as a treatment for diabetes – a work in progress. *N Engl J Med* 2004;350:694–705.

Sutherland DER, Gruessner RWG, Dunn DL et al. Lessons learned from more than 1000 pancreas transplants at a single institution. *Ann Surg* 2001;233:463–501.

Treatment of people with type 2 diabetes requires consideration of several aspects of the patient's health, and the range of areas is summarized in Table 7.1. Ideally, an individualized approach that considers the patient holistically is encouraged, with the patient becoming skilled in self-management of most aspects of their diabetes care. Each patient will have varying levels of diabetic complications, cardiovascular risk, risk from hypoglycemia and so on, and thus diabetes care should be tailored to individual needs.

It is important to consider care for the patient with type 2 diabetes from the perspective of a multidisciplinary team, with contributions from medical practitioners, nurse educators, dietitians and podiatrists. Psychologists can contribute substantially when appropriate.

At diagnosis, the patient should be given simple and clear messages about diabetes and how it may affect health with regard to complications and cardiovascular risk. Importantly, patients should be encouraged that, with excellent glucose, lipid and blood pressure control and smoking cessation, risks of complications and cardiovascular events can be reduced substantially.

Education

Education of the person with newly diagnosed type 2 diabetes is critical in helping them to take an active role in their own management. In this regard, the role of education is to inform and empower the individual, not merely tick off a checklist of complications and topics covered. For many people, the diagnosis of diabetes and the possibility of complications can be overwhelming, depressing and/or frightening. A sensitive approach, with interpretation of the patient's responses to each piece of information given, helps avoid the disempowerment, denial and fatalism that can be the response of some patients. A summary of areas to cover is provided in Table 7.2.

TABLE 7.1

Aspects of management

Diabetes education
- Establish an understanding of diet and physical activity therapy
- Where appropriate, encourage capillary blood glucose monitoring
- Footcare education
- Identification and treatment of hypoglycemia

Glycemic control to prevent diabetic complications
- Establish glycemic targets based on
  - HbA_{1c}
  - fasting and 2-hour postmeal glucose levels

Cardiovascular risk reduction
- Smoking cessation
- Lipid treatment to achieve target levels for primary and secondary prevention
- Hypertension control to normal range

Routine complication screening
- Annual retinal examinations, with an ophthalmologist check biennially
- Annual foot examination
- Annual microalbuminuria testing

Appropriate strategies to reduce weight if obesity present

Identify and treat sleep apnea

Identify and treat mood disorders, if present

Group education with discussion is often helpful and written information is useful as a record for the patient and to reinforce the information given verbally. Printed educational resources are often available from national diabetes patient advocacy and support bodies. Patients should be taught how to measure capillary blood glucose so they can monitor their control and detect and treat hyperglycemia.

TABLE 7.2

Areas to cover in diabetes education

- What is type 2 diabetes?
- Why does it develop?
- What problems can occur in diabetes?
- How do we prevent these from occurring?
- How do we monitor blood glucose?
- What is hypoglycemia?
- What does hypoglycemia feel like?
- How do we treat hypoglycemia?
- How do we look after our feet?
- When do I need to see my doctor quickly?

Foot self-care education is critical and includes care for feet, avoiding and treating fungal infection and avoiding foot injury from ill-fitting shoes, thermal trauma and barefoot walking. Care following minor trauma should be discussed. The individual should be encouraged to see a doctor for early intervention, as a small foot blister can rapidly turn into an infected ulcer and osteomyelitis.

Clinical assessment

The fundamentals of history and examination are critical in assessment for clinical comorbidities. Are there any clues to indicate the duration of diabetes? If present, when did the symptoms of hyperglycemia start? These signals may be as simple as fatigue or sleepiness after eating. Studies show type 2 diabetes is often present for 5 years prior to diagnosis. A family history of diabetic complications or heart disease is useful, as this may signpost a genetic predisposition to nephropathy or cardiovascular disease that helps identify patients for more aggressive prevention (for example, blood pressure normalization and excellent glucose and lipid control in those with a family history of diabetic nephropathy with chronic renal failure). A prior history or family history of myocardial infarction or heart disease mandates therapeutic targets of perfect lipids and blood pressure control, together with acetylsalicylic acid (ASA; aspirin) or anticoagulant as required.

Physical examination should identify the presence of overweight or obesity, central obesity (by waist measurement), hypertension, retinopathy and peripheral neuropathy. Signs of chronic liver disease should signal other possible diseases, such as hemochromatosis or advanced fatty liver disease. Signs of Cushing's syndrome or acromegaly should be sought.

Diet and exercise

Dietary intervention and increased physical activity are the cornerstones of management in the patient with diabetes and are discussed in detail in chapter 8.

Glycemic targets

A patient diagnosed with diabetes requires follow-up to determine whether diet, physical activity interventions and exercise and, where necessary, weight loss have sufficiently controlled capillary glucose levels and achieved optimal levels of glycated hemoglobin (HbA_{1c}). When glucose levels are in the teens or above, this follow-up period may be a couple of days; where blood glucose levels have been under 10 mmol/L (180 mg/dL), 1–2 months may be sufficient. If fasting glucose levels remain above 7.0 mmol/L (126 mg/dL) or postmeal glucose levels are above 10 mmol/L (180 mg/dL), drug therapy is indicated.

Over the longer term, HbA_{1c} levels can be used to measure whether glycemic control is acceptable. Generally, a target of HbA_{1c} between 6.0% and 7.0% (42 and 53 mmol/mol) is considered adequate control. There has been significant debate as to how tight glycemic control should be in type 2 diabetes, based on large studies such as the UK Prospective Diabetes Study (UKPDS) and intervention studies such as Action in Diabetes and Vascular Disease (ADVANCE) and Action to Control Cardiovascular Risk in Diabetes (ACCORD). While consensus has not been reached, a sensible approach is to consider the individual patients and their unique health needs but with an overall aim of reaching an HbA_{1c} below 7.0% (53 mmol/mol). In patients who are at risk of hypoglycemia, such as the elderly, a reasonable HbA_{1c} target is 6.5–7.0% (48–53 mmol/mol).

Drug therapy

If glucose monitoring or HbA_{1c} levels indicate suboptimal control, drug therapy needs to be considered. Drugs currently available to treat type 2 diabetes are listed in Table 7.3.

Metformin is a biguanide drug that is usually considered as a first-line agent in type 2 diabetes mellitus. It has several actions that promote glucose lowering. It is a modest insulin sensitizer that acts through improving post-insulin receptor signaling, promoting glucose uptake

TABLE 7.3

Medications currently available

Biguanides	Sulfonylureas	α-Glucosidase inhibitors
• Metformin	• Gliclazide	• Acarbose
	• Glibenclamide/ glyburide	
	• Glipizide	
	• Glimepiride	

Thiazoledinediones	Incretin therapy	Insulins
• Rosiglitazone	*DPP4 inhibitors*	• Very quick acting
• Pioglitazone	• Sitagliptin	• Quick acting
	• Vildagliptin	• Intermediate
	• Saxagliptin	• Long acting
	• Linagliptin	
	GLP-1 analogs	
	• Exenatide	
	• Liguratide	

DPP4, dipeptidyl peptidase-4; GLP-1, glucagon-like peptide-1.

in muscle and reducing hepatic glucose output. In this regard, it is quite useful in obese or overweight patients with higher fasting glucose levels when given at the evening meal. Metformin may also reduce appetite in some patients, which helps with weight reduction; this action is being studied.

Metformin can be administered once, twice or three times daily, either before or after the meal. Adverse effects can include nausea (hence taken after the meal), abdominal cramping or diarrhea. Dosing should start low (for example, 250 mg twice daily) and gradually increase over 2–4 weeks. For patients experiencing adverse effects, the dose should be halved and lowered further if symptoms do not resolve. An extended-release preparation may help avoid adverse effects.

Metformin doses should be lowered in renal disease. It should be avoided in patients with raised creatinine and heart failure as it can precipitate lactic acidosis.

Sulfonylureas are potent drugs that stimulate insulin secretion from the β cell by acting at a specific receptor. They can be given once or twice daily and extended-release forms are also available. A low dose can be started before the period in which the risk of hyperglycemia is greatest. For example, if there is fasting hyperglycemia, the sulfonylurea can be given before dinner; if there is daytime postprandial hyperglycemia, the sulfonylurea can be given at breakfast. Ideally, sulfonylureas are given 20–30 minutes before the meal.

Patients receiving sulfonylureas require education about hypoglycemia, which can be severe in some people. Patients need to be warned not to skip meals if they have taken their sulfonylurea. Likewise, patients should be asked to report symptoms of hypoglycemia as dose reduction may be necessary. A further side effect of sulfonylurea therapy is weight gain.

Thiazoledinediones act by stimulating a transcriptional factor, peroxisomal proliferator receptor γ, resulting in at least several actions that improve insulin sensitivity and glucose control. The thiazoledinediones are generally given once or twice daily. Adverse effects include weight gain and fluid retention, which can precipitate cardiac failure in patients with underlying cardiac disease. There is also an increased risk of fracture. Most recently, some controversial data have suggested a potential increased risk of bladder cancer with prolonged use, though further data are awaited.

Incretin therapy refers to two classes of hypoglycemic agent that act by mimicking or increasing circulating levels of gut peptides such as glucagon-like peptide-1 (GLP-1). The GLP-1 analogs are considered to act directly on the β cells to stimulate insulin secretion; the dipeptidyl peptidase-4 (DPP4) inhibitors act by reducing breakdown of endogenous GLP-1, thereby boosting its systemic half-life and action.

α-Glucosidase inhibitors. The glucosidase inhibitor acarbose induces a modest reduction in postprandial glucose excursions by reducing dissacharide breakdown and monosaccharide absorption in the gut. Side effects include abdominal distention and flatus.

Insulin therapy (see Chapter 6) is frequently required in type 2 diabetes mellitus. The defect in type 2 diabetes is insufficient insulin production to meet demand. Studies indicate there is gradual decline of insulin production with time. A common clinical scenario over time is that patients treated with diet and exercise eventually slide away from the treatment targets they had achieved previously, oral drugs are added sequentially and, over the course of 10 years, the condition progresses, with further insulin deficiency and drug refractoriness, such that insulin replacement therapy becomes necessary.

In type 2 diabetes, insulin can be given as a long-acting single dose before bedtime. The aim is to normalize fasting glucose. Other drugs such as metformin and sulfonylureas are continued. Other dosing regimens include twice daily premixed insulin for older patients or a basal–bolus regimen for patients who can manage a more complex insulin dosing regimen.

Patient monitoring will indicate the success of insulin addition. If there is significant postmeal glucose excursion (despite dietetic intervention), preprandial short-acting insulin may become necessary.

Care should be taken to ensure patients are well educated in hypoglycemia detection and treatment and that overnight hypoglycemia does not occur. This is a particular issue in older patients who have underlying cardiovascular and cerebrovascular disease.

Weight reduction and bariatric surgery

In obese patients with type 2 diabetes, consideration should be given to obesity-management strategies, including bariatric surgery (see chapter 8). Modest weight reduction of 5 kg can significantly improve glucose control, in addition to benefitting other metabolic factors that accompany diabetes, including hyperlipidemia, hypertension, sleep apnea and non-alcoholic liver disease. Again, diet and exercise play a critical role and are discussed in detail in chapter 8. Also see *Fast Facts: Obesity*.

Other management targets

Smoking cessation is critical in reducing macrovascular disease in patients with diabetes. Patients who smoke should be supported with psychological strategies and, where appropriate, drug therapy to stop smoking. See *Fast Facts: Smoking Cessation*.

Hypertension. Blood pressure should ideally be normalized in patients with diabetes. Weight reduction and increased physical activity may have some benefit; multiple drugs are often necessary. A target of 120/80 mmHg is appropriate, even lower in those with microalbuminuria. See *Fast Facts: Hypertension*.

Lipid-lowering therapy. People with type 2 diabetes have a risk of a cardiac event that is equal to that of people with a prior myocardial infarct. Risk reduction includes lifestyle management (including diet, weight loss, exercise, smoking cessation and blood pressure control). Lipid-lowering therapy is often indicated. Statin therapy is indicated if the total cholesterol exceeds 5.0 mmol/L (193 mg/dL). Fibrate therapy is indicated in those patients with predominant hypertriglyceridemia for whom lifestyle modification has not normalized triglyceride levels. See *Fast Facts: Hyperlipidemia*.

ASA (aspirin) at a low dose should be considered in all patients with type 2 diabetes for its cardioprotective effects.

Key points – treatment of type 2 diabetes mellitus

- Type 2 diabetes management requires patient education on the fundamentals of self-care, including monitoring of glucose levels, dietary management – with an emphasis on weight reduction in the overweight or obese – increased physical activity and reduced sedentariness.
- Medications are often required for glucose control, including metformin, sulfonylureas, thiazolidinediones and insulin, in addition to newer agents such as the glucagon-like peptide-1 (GLP-1) agonists and dipeptidyl peptidase-4 (DPP4) inhibitors.
- Glycemic treatment targets aim for an HbA$_{1c}$ that ranges from 6.0% to 7.0%, depending on the age of the patients and their risk for hypoglycemia.
- All patients with type 2 diabetes who smoke must receive smoking cessation intervention(s).
- Cardiovascular risk factors must be treated to targets, including lipids and blood pressure. Consideration should be given to acetylsalicylic acid (ASA; aspirin) therapy where appropriate.
- Bariatric surgery should be considered in the obese with type 2 diabetes and poor glycemic control.

Key references

Bloomgarden ZT. Approaches to treatment of pre-diabetes and obesity and promising new approaches to type 2 diabetes. *Diabetes Care* 2008;31:1461–6.

LeRoith D. Treatment of diabetes: a clinical update on insulin trials. *Clin Cornerstone* 2007;8:21–9.

Salehi M, Aulinger BA, D'Alessio DA. Targeting beta-cell mass in type 2 diabetes: promise and limitations of new drugs based on incretins. *Endocr Rev* 2008;29:367–79.

Diet and physical activity

Principles of dietary management

Type 1 diabetes mellitus is characterized by absolute insulin deficiency and type 2 diabetes by insulin resistance and relative insulin deficiency. Thus, there is an inability of the body to produce sufficient insulin to meet requirements. Essentially, there are basal insulin requirements and additional insulin requirements determined by foods consumed, stress, illness and so on. Lipid disorders often accompany type 2 diabetes, and hypertension or renal disease may also require specific dietary instructions. Therefore, appropriate dietary advice in the patient with diabetes considers the individual patient's needs, both health and cultural (Table 8.1).

TABLE 8.1

Factors influencing nutritional advice

Factor	Issue	Strategy
Glycemic control	Not on target	Improve all aspects of diet
Weight	Overweight or obese	Reduce weight
Central obesity	Waist > 90 cm (men), > 86 cm (women)	Reduce weight
Hypoglycemia	Timing?	Adjust dose or snack
Renal failure		Consider protein intake
Hypertension	Controlled? Diuretics?	Consider salt intake
Medication type	Oral hypoglycemics or insulin?	
Vegetarian	Protein sufficient? Fat on target?	
Cultural preferences/ religion	Hypoglycemic risk if fasting?	Adjust dose

The fundamentals of diet in diabetes

Dietary recommendations for the last 30 years in diabetes mellitus have emphasized a diet low in saturated fat. Macronutrient breakdown consisted of less than 30% of energy intake from fat (with less than 10% from saturated sources), 50–60% of energy from carbohydrates and 20% from protein. The imperative for a low saturated fat intake in diabetes was (and still is) mandated by the need to limit dietary cholesterol and reduce cardiovascular risk.

Glycemic index. In the last two decades, the inclusion of foods with a 'low glycemic index' (GI) within the 50–60% carbohydrate component has been suggested. Low GI carbohydrates generally have a high fiber content, which apparently slows the absorption of glucose from the gut. Thus, in some patients, the postprandial glycemic excursion may be less exaggerated if carbohydrate choices have a low GI. There is great variability in the individual response to 'low GI' foods, however. Some low GI foods may be helpful in preventing between meal hypoglycemia, particularly in those patients using isophane and short-acting insulins. However, overconsumption of even high-quality low GI foods can lead to postprandial hyperglycemia and weight gain. Thus, as in all food groups, quantity matters.

Balance of macronutrients. More recently, it has been accepted that different dietary approaches are also appropriate in type 2 diabetes. Specifically, accepted macronutrient content has become more flexible.

The first change was the acceptance that different types of fats were not necessarily as harmful as saturated fat. Studies have shown that a higher intake of fat from monounsaturated fat sources improves the glycemic and lipid profiles. Sources of monounsaturated fats include olive and canola oil, avocados and some nuts. Individual need should be considered again: if obesity is an issue and weight loss is desired, energy intake reduction may be compromised if there is increased energy intake by increased consumption of fat, even if it is of high quality.

The second change has been the acceptance that lower carbohydrate and higher protein intakes are acceptable and beneficial in type 2 diabetes. Protein sources should remain low in saturated fat. In the patient with excellent or tight glycemic control, insulin or hypoglycemic drugs may require dose reduction with carbohydrate intake reduction, particularly if omitted from any particular meal.

Several studies have now shown certain nutrients, including fish oils and monounsaturated fats in the form of olive oil, have cardioprotective effects in people with heart disease. While such studies have not been performed specifically in people with diabetes, it would nevertheless seem prudent to advise that people with diabetes add fish-based meals to their diet and use olive oil as the main oil or fat in the diet.

Thus, dietary intake in type 2 diabetes can be flexible in macronutrient intake; the emphasis on a low intake of saturated animal and vegetable fats remains.

Diet in insulin-treated patients

Insulin-treated patients (type 1 or type 2 diabetes) receiving meal-time quick-acting insulin (either singly or in a premixed form) need to eat carbohydrate at that meal. It is useful to refer to standard portion sizes or exchanges of carbohydrates for patients, and ensure the premeal insulin dose covers the carbohydrate sufficiently to prevent postmeal hyperglycemia or hypoglycemia. Postmeal glucose testing can help to determine the appropriate premeal insulin dose. It is outside the scope of this chapter to discuss carbohydrate portion size extensively. Patients treated with premeal insulin should receive specific counseling from a dietitian skilled in management of insulin-treated patients.

Further, insulin-treated patients may be at risk of hypoglycemia. This occurs more commonly with isophane insulins (with which the hypoglycemia can occur overnight or between meals) or following meals after short-acting insulin. Between-meal and overnight hypoglycemia may occur less frequently with some of the newer insulins, such as the very-long-acting insulins or the very-quick-acting insulins. Nevertheless, some patients will need to consume a snack, such as a glass of milk or a piece of fruit, at bedtime to prevent overnight hypoglycemia; other times of risk are mid morning or afternoon. Care needs to be exercised not to increase total energy intake substantially, otherwise weight gain may occur. If hypoglycemia regularly occurs at the same time, it would be reasonable to reduce the preceding dose of insulin or, if possible, consider changing the insulin type.

Weight loss

A desire to lose weight is common in many patients with type 2 diabetes. This area can be particularly challenging when overweight or obese patients have gained more weight as a consequence of their therapies – sulfonylureas, thiazolidinediones and insulin can promote weight gain.

There are numerous weight-loss approaches for obese patients with diabetes. The evidence does not suggest that one approach is better than any other; the key element for successful weight loss is enduring and consistent energy restriction.

Energy restriction. Simple approaches for energy restriction revolve around reducing consumption of energy-dense foods, making informed choices through reading food labels and reducing meal sizes.

Reduce energy-dense foods. Simple instructions to limit the most energy-dense foods – usually those containing high concentrations of fats and/or simple sugars, such as convenience or takeaway foods – often result in energy restriction. More frequently, foods claiming to be 'low fat', 'light' or '99% fat free' can have a high content of added simple or complex sugars. These can undermine a patient's attempts to restrict energy intake and may worsen their glucose control.

Food labels will indicate to patients the total energy, fat and carbohydrate content of any particular food. They are found on most foods, depending on laws within individual countries. Patients may need support to interpret food labels and identify energy-dense foods. By acquiring knowledge of food labels and composition, healthcare professionals can help patients navigate this potentially confusing area. There are many small detailed handbooks on the energy and nutrient composition of foods that can help professionals and patients select low-energy items.

Recent trends in foods available in supermarkets have included the addition of carbohydrates derived from fruits or other sources, which are added to improve the palatability of food. These might be labeled as 'natural fruit juice', fructose, corn or maize starch, to name a few. These additions increase the energy density of the food and again can undermine energy restriction targets and glucose control.

Reduction of meal size is a further simple instruction to reduce energy intake. Another useful strategy is reducing or restricting between-meal snacks in those patients not at risk of hypoglycemia.

Avoiding hypoglycemia. With energy restriction, the potential for hypoglycemia with the patient's drug therapy should be considered. Patients treated with sulfonylureas or insulin are at risk and may require dose reduction when undertaking energy restriction. Patients treated with single drugs that do not induce hypoglycemia (metformin, acarbose, thiazolidinediones, sitagliptin) do not require dose reduction.

Very low energy diets. In selected patients, replacement of one, two or all meals with a protein-based shake is also feasible and will result in significant energy restriction. Programs using this approach have been found to be successful and safe in the longer term. Many products are available from a variety of commercial sources. These products can be diverse in their energy and sugar content and vary between 140 and 200 kcal (560–800 kJ) per serving; some are even higher. When suggesting any product, the health professional will need to consider whether the product contains the daily requirement of vitamins and minerals; if not, vitamin supplements should be recommended.

The doses of hypoglycemic agents and insulin should be reduced when starting this form of eating plan (by 30–50%), and the patient should be warned that hypoglycemia may still develop; further reductions in medication are often required, generally within 1–4 weeks. With prolonged use (longer than 12 weeks) iron and vitamin B_{12} levels should be checked.

Bariatric surgery in type 2 diabetes. Recent studies indicate that weight loss with the aid of bariatric surgery will restore glucose metabolism.

The Swedish Obesity Study found 98% of diabetic participants had normalized glucose levels at 2 years following a number of surgical procedures, including gastric banding, sleeve gastrectomy, vertical gastroplasty and Roux-en-Y gastric bypass. More recently, gastric banding plus a supported lifestyle program was found to normalize glucose metabolism in 75% of subjects at 2 years. It is important to note that studies of bariatric surgery in type 2 diabetes were performed in centers expert in bariatric surgery and that patients were intensively supported by a multidisciplinary team. Centers offering surgery without this or patients reluctant to participate in follow-up may not reach these levels of success.

Bariatric surgery may be suitable for the obese patient with type 2 diabetes, particularly if other obesity comorbidities exist. Patients benefit from support from an expert in the specific dietary requirements following bariatric surgery. Again, because of the energy restriction that occurs after surgery, adjustment of hypoglycemic agents is necessary.

Physical activity

Increasing physical activity is a cornerstone in the management of diabetes mellitus. It improves the action of insulin, reduces blood pressure, improves the lipid profile and can reduce the risk of heart disease and stroke. Physical activity is also essential in strategies to maintain or reduce weight.

It is recommended that people with diabetes exercise for 20 minutes three days per week, at an intensity of 50% VO_2 max (i.e. 50% of maximal aerobic capacity). This is generally at a level where, during the exercise, a person would be able to talk in short sentences only.

If there are weight issues, patients should be encouraged to exercise on a daily basis, with sessions of longer duration and lower intensity than described above. A prescription of 40 minutes of walking per day is reasonable, to be accrued over several sessions. This may be particularly suitable for older patients and those with degenerative joint disease, heart disease, neuropathy or physical disability – conditions that can make longer exercise episodes problematic.

Pedometers are useful for encouraging patients and tracking activity; patients can be encouraged to build up to 10 000 steps daily. This needs to be tempered by consideration of physical disability and underlying fitness. It is generally wise to encourage a gradual build up for those who have been sedentary for a long time. Encourage patients with cardiac disease to build up their exercise level gradually, starting with walking.

Patients with renal failure, microalbuminuria or retinopathy should be discouraged from participating in physical activity that could raise blood pressure significantly. This might include weight lifting and 'burst' anaerobic sports.

All patients with diabetes should be encouraged to wear comfortable flexible-soled shoes with good arch support. Patients with neuropathy should be encouraged to check their feet after exercise and treat blisters if detected. Exercising barefoot should be discouraged, particularly for those with neuropathy.

As exercise improves insulin action, hypoglycemia may occur after exercise. This effect can occur immediately, but may last for 24 hours after the exercise bout. Therefore, insulin-treated patients may need to reduce insulin doses for subsequent meals and even the overnight long-acting insulin dose. Some patients may reduce insulin doses prior to the planned exercise too.

Patients should be encouraged to monitor glucose levels after exercise and snack as necessary. Some patients may need a carbohydrate snack prior to the exercise bout. For prolonged exercise, such as long walks, golf and other activities, snacks may be needed during the exercise too. Strategies for avoiding hypoglycemia in exercise are summarized in Table 8.2.

TABLE 8.2

Strategies for avoiding hypoglycemia with exercise

- Consume carbohydrate snack before exercise
- Reduce insulin dose before exercise
- Reduce subsequent insulin doses
- Snack during exercise

Key points – diet and physical activity

- Diet for healthy weight and optimized glucose control is one of the cornerstones of diabetes self-care.
- Increased physical activity and reduced sedentariness are fundamental to physical health and healthy weight in diabetes control.
- Suitable management plans for people with diabetes will include addressing nutrition and physical activity, using the skill sets of allied health professionals including dietitians and exercise physiologists, where available. If these specialists are not available or easily accessible, others involved in patient care, including general practitioners, diabetes educators and endocrinologists are ideally placed to provide lifestyle advice to people with diabetes.

Key reference

American Diabetes Association.
Standards of care. *Diabetes Care*
2011;34(suppl 1):S16–27.

On a population basis, most deaths and morbidity stem from the development of the chronic complications of diabetes, despite the fact that deaths continue to occur as a consequence of hypoglycemia and diabetic ketoacidosis. It is the symptoms that arise from the many complications of diabetes and the psychological effects of the condition itself that seriously impact on quality of life.

Around 20% of people with type 2 diabetes have at least one identifiable complication at the time of diagnosis, largely because of the long delay between the onset of diabetes and its final diagnosis. Many patients will, however, live without a significant burden of symptomatic diabetes complications. The chronic complications of diabetes mellitus are shown in Table 9.1. The time and financial resources spent on screening, detecting and managing chronic complications of diabetes are substantial.

TABLE 9.1

Complications of diabetes

Acute

- Hypoglycemia
- Diabetic ketoacidosis
- Hyperosmolar hyperglycemic state

Chronic

Microvascular complications	*Macrovascular complications*
• Neuropathy	• Hypertension
• Retinopathy	• Cardiovascular disease
• Nephropathy	• Cerebrovascular disease
• Diabetic foot	• Peripheral vascular disease
	• Erectile dysfunction

Diabetic neuropathy

Neuropathy in diabetes is common and may have many and varied manifestations. The types of neuropathy seen in diabetic patients are set out in Table 9.2. The risk of developing neuropathy is directly linked to the duration of diabetes: after 20 years of diabetes, about 40% of patients have neuropathy (though equally, and interestingly, some 60% will not). The precise cause of diabetic neuropathy has not been identified. There seems no doubt that it is related to hyperglycemia, with the possibility of mild neuropathy associated with impaired glucose tolerance being present before the development of frank diabetes.

The involvement of small nerve fibers is the earliest detectable sign of neuropathy. Accumulation of polyols and the formation of advanced glycation endproducts are possible factors in the etiology of diabetic neuropathy and an increasing body of evidence supports a role for oxidative stress. Ischemia is also likely to be involved in the development of diabetic nerve damage and again there is some evidence to support this.

Chronic insidious sensorimotor neuropathy, often accompanied by asymptomatic motor impairment, is the most frequent abnormality of nerve function seen in diabetes. It may be present at the time of first diagnosis in patients with type 2 diabetes, reflecting the duration of the disorder before formal detection. Patients may have few symptoms or complain of paresthesias, numbness, discomfort or pain

TABLE 9.2

Neuropathy in diabetes

- Chronic insidious sensorimotor neuropathy
- Acute painful neuropathy
- Proximal motor neuropathy
- Diabetic mononeuropathy
- Diabetic autonomic neuropathy

accompanied by demonstrable distal sensory loss, loss of vibration sense and loss of deep-tendon reflexes. Motor nerves tend to be affected later, which may result in distal weakness and atrophy, though this is much less common than the sensory symptoms. Once established, this type of neuropathy is usually resistant to treatment other than the use of drugs for symptomatic pain relief. Aside from the unpleasant symptoms, the significance of this type of neuropathy is that once severe, sensory loss – together with lower-limb ischemia – becomes a major risk factor for the development of neuropathic ulceration and a Charçot joint.

Acute painful neuropathy. Fortunately, this type of neuropathy is relatively uncommon. It is associated with severe pain in the thighs, legs and feet, which may be excruciating and completely disabling, with attendant muscle weakness and wasting. Acute painful neuropathy is usually seen in the context of poor glycemic control, but it may emerge during a period of rapid improvement in control. Smoking and excess alcohol intake are associated with more severe symptoms in patients with painful diabetic neuropathy (PDN). Fortunately, most individuals recover spontaneously within a year. Good glycemic control is important to achieve this.

Proximal motor neuropathy (diabetic amyotrophy) is sometimes referred to as Garland's syndrome or diabetic femoral neuropathy, though the latter term is not an accurate reflection of the putative pathophysiology. The term 'diabetic lumbosacral plexopathy' has been proposed as, though the exact pathogenesis remains to be determined, most authors now favor an immune vasculopathy (inflammatory immune-mediated vascular radiculoplexopathy) as the most likely cause of diabetic amyotrophy. Fortunately it is rare, with an overall prevalence of around 0.08% in patients with diabetes.

Diabetic amyotrophy is most common in patients over the age of 50 years. The onset is usually gradual but it may, in certain cases, be abrupt. The initial symptom is asymmetric pain in the hip, buttock or thigh, which is followed by proximal weakness of the lower-limb muscles. Occasionally the symptoms are unilateral. Diabetic amyotrophy usually occurs in the context of poor blood glucose control. An interesting and frequently reported feature of amyotrophy is weight loss. Sometimes the symptoms are so severe that they lead to depression requiring treatment.

Physical examination reveals proximal lower-limb weakness with wasting associated with minimal sensory loss (Figure 9.1). Characteristically, the patient has difficulty getting up from a squatting position. Knee-jerk reflexes are absent but ankle reflexes may be present unless there is an accompanying distal neuropathy. Electrophysiological studies reveal a lumbosacral plexopathy.

Recovery from diabetic amyotrophy is slow. The establishment of good glycemic control, usually with insulin treatment, is paramount.

Physiotherapy is helpful. Tricyclic antidepressants may help alleviate both the pain and the depression associated with this condition. Duloxetine, gabapentin and pregabalin may also provide pain relief. Other treatments used for diabetic lumbosacral plexopathy are intravenous human immunoglobulin, cyclophosphamide and methylprednisolone, though proven benefit has yet to be established in controlled studies.

Diabetic mononeuropathy. Neuropathies affecting single nerves or their roots are common in diabetes. Such mononeuropathies are usually of rapid onset and severe in nature, though most affected individuals recover with time. Mononeuropathies affect the cranial or peripheral nerves. Third cranial nerve palsies are relatively common in diabetes (Figure 9.2), while fourth and sixth cranial nerve palsies

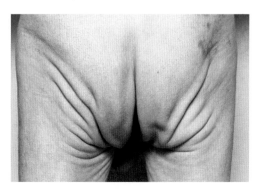

Figure 9.1 Diabetic neuropathy presenting as amyotrophy, with wasting of the thigh and glutei muscles.

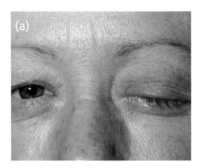
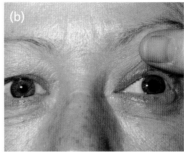

Figure 9.2 Right third cranial nerve palsy. (a) The patient cannot open the left eye due to complete left ptosis. (b) When the eyelid is lifted the eye is found to be turned out, in this case with a dilated pupil. Reproduced courtesy of Dr Anthony Pane, Mater Hospital, Brisbane, Australia.

(Figure 9.3) also occur. These palsies are thought to have a vascular etiology. Pressure palsies are common and typically involve the median nerve, resulting in classic carpal tunnel syndrome. Ulnar and sciatic nerve palsies (common peroneal, lateral popliteal) are also seen. Lateral popliteal nerve palsy may cause foot drop. Where more than one nerve is involved, a mononeuritis multiplex picture develops. Truncal neuropathy presents with acute onset of pain in the distribution of a truncal nerve mimicking herpes zoster; it may be seen in association with mononeuritis multiplex or it can occur in isolation.

Diabetic autonomic neuropathy. Abnormal tests of autonomic function are frequently found in diabetic patients, particularly in those with clinical evidence of sensory neuropathy. However, symptoms

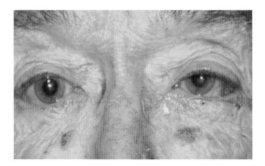

Figure 9.3 Left sixth cranial nerve palsy. Reproduced courtesy of Dr William Campbell, Royal Victorian Eye and Ear Hospital, Melbourne, Australia.

attributable to autonomic neuropathy are uncommon and are usually seen in those patients with a history of longstanding poorly controlled type 1 diabetes. Autonomic neuropathy, when it affects the cardiovascular system, is relatively easy to detect using simple tests such as assessing the heart rate response to the Valsalva maneuver, deep breathing and moving from the supine to the erect posture. The normally increased variation in heart rate during deep breathing is not observed in autonomic neuropathy. The blood pressure response to sustained hand grip and standing up can also be studied. A fall in blood pressure of more than 30 mmHg on standing suggests severe peripheral sympathetic damage, as does an increase in blood pressure of less than 10 mmHg during sustained handgrip (30% of maximum handgrip as determined using a hand grip dynamometer sustained for as long as possible up to 5 minutes). Evaluating autonomic function in other systems is much more complicated and is not routinely carried out in clinical practice.

Table 9.3 lists how autonomic neuropathy may affect the diabetic patient. Diabetic autonomic neuropathy, when symptomatic and not just detected by abnormal tests on autonomic function, is often associated with a poor long-term outlook.

Abnormal sweating is seen as a manifestation of autonomic neuropathy. Gustatory sweating occurs in response to eating certain foods and is associated with profuse sweating affecting the face and upper chest.

Postural hypotension occurs as a consequence of sympathetic denervation and may be very troublesome and refractory to treatment.

Gastrointestinal effects. Vagal denervation of the stomach results in diabetic gastroparesis, which wreaks havoc in the control of type 1 diabetes because of delayed and variable gastric emptying. Diabetic diarrhea may result from abnormal gut motility caused by autonomic denervation (perhaps compounded by bacterial overgrowth). It is relatively uncommon, runs a variable course and is often nocturnal in nature. Diabetic constipation is also seen.

Genitourinary effects. The diabetic neuropathic bladder produces bladder dysfunction secondary to autonomic neuropathy affecting the

TABLE 9.3

Clinical features of diabetic autonomic neuropathy

Sudomotor
- Gustatory sweating
- Diabetic anhydrosis

Pupillary abnormalities
- Reduced resting diameter
- Delayed or absent response to light
- Diminished hippus

Cardiovascular
- Postural hypotension
- Resting tachycardia
- Loss of heart rate variation
- Painless myocardial infarction

Gastrointestinal
- Impaired esophageal motility
- Diarrhea
- Gastric atony
- Colonic atony
- Enlarged gallbladder

Respiratory
- Respiratory arrest

Urogenital
- Bladder dysfunction
- Retrograde ejaculation
- Impotence
- Loss of testicular sensation

Vasomotor
- Loss of skin vasomotor responses
- Edema

sacral nerves. Bladder emptying is impaired leading to a distended bladder and overflow incontinence.

Autonomic neuropathy may cause erectile dysfunction, although failure of erection in diabetic patients is now thought largely to be due to underlying vascular disease.

Treatment of diabetic autonomic neuropathy usually proves to be a challenge. Postural hypotension may respond to fludrocortisone, 0.1–0.5 mg daily. Prokinetic agents used to treat gastroparesis include metoclopramide, domperidone, erythromycin and levosulpiride. Intractable cases have been treated by gastric electrical stimulation using an implantable neurostimulator. Diabetic diarrhea may improve with the use of colestyramine, a somatostatin analog, pancreatic enzyme supplements or antibiotics such as metronidazole.

Sudden death is described in patients with severe autonomic neuropathy.

Pain should be treated with simple analgesics at first. When these fail to control neuropathic pain, other agents can be tried. The American Academy of Neurology has examined the evidence base for the treatment of PDN. Pregabalin was deemed to be the only drug with the strongest level of evidence to show that it can reduce pain in PDN. Less strong evidence supported the use of gabapentin, sodium valproate, duloxetine, amitriptyline and venlafaxine. Other drugs used in the treatment of PDN include carbamazepine, phenytoin, lamotrigine and topiramate.

On these grounds many guidelines suggest the use of pregabalin as a first-line agent for the treatment of PDN, and if this fails to try a tricyclic antidepressant or duloxetine before moving on to the other agents if they fail to be effective. None of these drugs will provide complete relief from PDN: the expected improvement is in the range 30–50%. Lidocaine (lignocaine) and tramadol can be used to treat painful neuropathy, although it is best to avoid opioid use where possible.

Non-pharmacological treatments include nerve-stimulation therapies and electrical spinal-cord stimulation. Capsaicin cream, which depletes axonal neuropeptide substance P, may occasionally help neuropathic pain.

Diabetic retinopathy

The prevalence of diabetic retinopathy increases with the duration of diabetes. Patients with type 1 diabetes do not exhibit retinopathy at the time of diagnosis, whereas retinopathy may be present at the time of diagnosis of type 2 diabetes, reflecting the fact that the diagnosis of diabetes has escaped recognition for some years. The majority (80–90%) of patients show some degree of retinopathy after

20 years of diabetes. Visual loss usually results from proliferative retinopathy in type 1 diabetes and from maculopathy in type 2 diabetes. Diabetes is the most common cause of blindness in people aged 20–60 years in western countries.

A classification of diabetic retinopathy is shown in Table 9.4. The first detectable abnormality is capillary dilatation, partly caused by an increase in retinal blood flow. Later features of a background diabetic retinopathy are microaneurysms, blot hemorrhages and hard exudates (Figure 9.4). Microaneurysms are localized capillary dilatations caused by pericyte loss. Ruptured microaneurysms result in retinal hemorrhages either superficially (flame-shaped hemorrhages) or in deeper layers of the retina (blot and dot hemorrhages). Capillary leakage of lipids and proteins results in exudate formation. Background non-proliferative retinopathy is not associated with visual loss.

Preproliferative retinopathy is indicated by the presence of cotton-wool spots (soft exudates), venous loops, arterial narrowing and occlusion, and intraretinal microvascular abnormalities (IRMAs) (Figure 9.5). Cotton-wool spots represent infarction of the nerve fiber layer from occlusion of precapillary arterioles. Venous loops reflect increasing retinal ischemia and are the most significant predictor of progression to proliferative retinopathy. IRMAs occur in areas of widespread capillary occlusion and consist of remodeled dilated abnormal capillary beds. Marked caliber variation of arteries precedes arterial occlusion which, if it occurs rapidly, produces cotton-wool spots. If the preproliferative state is recognized, the patient should be urgently referred to an ophthalmologist or vitreoretinal surgeon.

Further increases in retinal ischemia trigger the production of various vasoproliferative factors, such as vascular endothelial growth factor (VEGF), that stimulate new vessel formation; this is 'proliferative diabetic retinopathy' (Figures 9.6 and 9.7).

New vessels originate from major veins (occasionally from arteries) and most commonly occur near the optic disc (neovascularization of the disc) or within disc diameters of major retinal vessels (peripheral neovascularization). New vessels are fragile and are disrupted easily by vitreous traction, leading to hemorrhage into the vitreous cavity

TABLE 9.4

Classification of diabetic retinopathy and the associated ophthalmic changes

Background (simple) retinopathy

- Microaneurysms
- Hemorrhages (macula not involved)
- Hard exudates

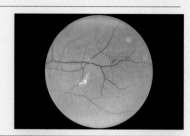

Preproliferative retinopathy

- Soft exudates (see right)
- Intraretinal microvascular abnormalities
- Venous abnormalities

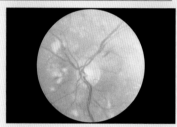

Proliferative retinopathy

- New vessel formation
- Vitreous hemorrhage
- Rubeosis iridis and secondary glaucoma may be complications

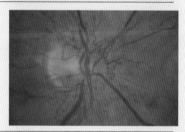

Maculopathy

- Multiple small hemorrhages around the macula (diffuse hemorrhagic maculopathy)
- Hard exudates around the macula (focal exudative maculopathy – see right)

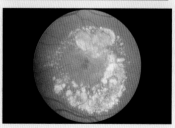

- Appearance may be normal, but vision impaired because of edema or ischemia (diffuse edematous or ischemic maculopathy)

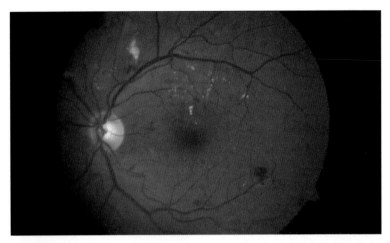

Figure 9.4 Background diabetic retinopathy. The microaneurysms are seen as scattered red spots. They are smaller and rounder than the blot hemorrhages, which have less distinct borders. The hard exudates appear as yellow or white areas. Reproduced courtesy of Dr William Campbell, Royal Victorian Eye and Ear Hospital, Melbourne, Australia.

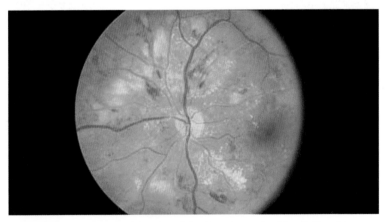

Figure 9.5 Severe preproliferative diabetic retinopathy. The fluffy white patches known as cotton-wool spots (soft exudates) are clearly visible.

(Figure 9.8a) or the preretinal space, resulting in sudden devastating visual loss. New vessels are also associated with fibroglial tissue (Figures 9.8b and c) which, when it contracts, may cause tractional retinal detachment with loss of vision that may be profound if it

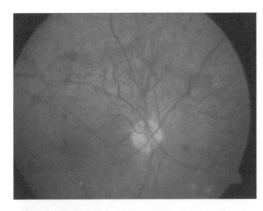

Figure 9.6 Proliferative diabetic retinopathy, with new vessel formation on the retinal surface. Reproduced courtesy of Dr William Campbell, Royal Victorian Eye and Ear Hospital, Melbourne, Australia.

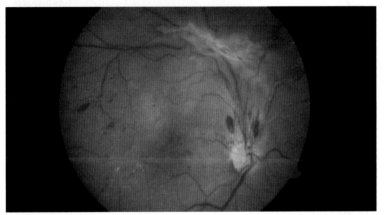

Figure 9.7 Late-stage proliferative diabetic retinopathy. Fibrous tissue (white area) is gathering around new vessels. Reproduced courtesy of Dr William Campbell, Royal Victorian Eye and Ear Hospital, Melbourne, Australia.

affects the macula. Rubeosis iridis (Figure 9.8d) occurs when new vessel formation spreads to affect the iris – it may cause secondary glaucoma and is a very serious eye condition.

Diabetic maculopathy, though not uncommon in type 1 diabetes, is much more commonly seen in type 2 diabetes (Figure 9.9). The most common form is exudative maculopathy: hard exudate rings form, usually lateral to the foveal area, and gradually approach the fovea. Another common form is edematous maculopathy, consisting of widespread and often cystic edema. The third form of maculopathy is

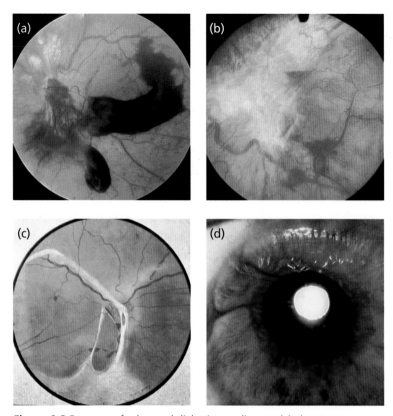

Figure 9.8 Features of advanced diabetic eye disease: (a) vitreous hemorrhage; (b) pre-retinal fibrosis and neovascularization; (c) traction vitreous bands; and (d) rubeosis iridis.

ischemic maculopathy in which perifoveal capillaries are destroyed. The fovea is located in the center of the macula and is responsible for central vision. Diabetic maculopathy is the most common cause of visual loss in diabetes, with ischemic maculopathy having the worst prognosis for vision.

Screening and referral. All patients with diabetes must be screened at least annually for the presence of diabetic retinopathy. In many countries, this is done by digital retinal photography with images graded by a retinal screener and abnormal retinal images being

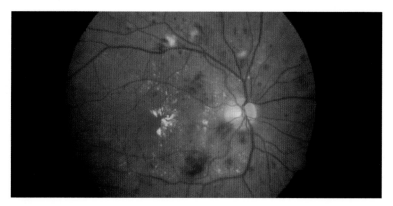

Figure 9.9 Diabetic maculopathy. This patient has clinically significant macular edema with adjacent hard exudates. The microaneurysms and hemorrhages are typical of focal maculopathy. Reproduced courtesy of Dr William Campbell, Royal Victorian Eye and Ear Hospital, Melbourne, Australia.

reviewed by an ophthalmologist. Criteria for referral to a specialist eye service are listed in Table 9.5.

Treatment. Laser photocoagulation is used to treat proliferative diabetic retinopathy and maculopathy (Figure 9.10). New vessels are photocoagulated and, in cases of more severe proliferative retinopathy, panretinal photocoagulation is performed (i.e. laser burns to the entire retina, sparing the central macular area). The strategy for treating macular edema depends on the type and extent of vessel leakage. With focal leakage, microaneurysms are treated directly with laser photocoagulation. With non-specific foci of leakage, a grid of laser burns is applied. Photocoagulation aims to destroy hypoxic retinal tissue and may decrease the overproduction of vasoactive factors such as VEGF. Vitrectomy may be necessary to treat vitreous hemorrhage that fails to resolve spontaneously. Although not yet established as standard therapy, intravitreal injections of VEGF inhibitors – drugs used in the treatment of wet macular degeneration such as ranibizumab – have shown promise in the treatment of diabetic macular edema. Intraocular steroids are also used to treat this condition. ACE inhibitors may have a beneficial role in the treatment or prevention of diabetic retinopathy.

TABLE 9.5

Criteria for referral to an eye specialist

Immediate referral
- Vitreous hemorrhage
- Neovascular glaucoma

Referral within 1 week
- Fall in visual acuity of ≥ 2 lines on Snellen chart
- Established maculopathy (edema of macula, hard exudates on macula)
- New vessels at periphery or at optic disc
- Rubeosis iridis
- Advanced diabetic retinopathy (e.g. retinal detachment)

Non-urgent referral (within a few weeks)
- Hard exudates close to macula
- Florid and increasing number of retinal hemorrhages
- Preproliferative changes

Routine referral
- Cataract

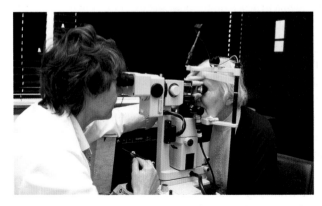

Figure 9.10 Diabetic retinopathy can be treated by photocoagulation using an argon laser.

Diabetic nephropathy

Diabetic nephropathy is characterized by persistent albuminuria (> 300 mg/day), decreasing glomerular filtration and increasing blood pressure in the context of diabetes and without other features to suggest glomerulonephritis. In the National Health and Nutrition Examination Survey (NHANES), the prevalence of diabetic kidney disease in the US population increased from 2.2% between 1988 and 1994 to 3.3% between 2005 and 2008. The prevalence increased in direct proportion to the prevalence of diabetes mellitus in the population with no increase in prevalence in those with established diabetes.

Diabetic nephropathy has become the leading cause of chronic renal failure in the USA and other western societies. It accounts for 30–40% of cases of end-stage renal failure in the USA. Proteinuria occurs in 15–40% of patients with type 1 diabetes and rarely develops before 10 years' duration. In patients with type 2 diabetes the prevalence is highly variable, ranging from 5% to 20%. Nephropathy is frequently associated with the development of type 1 diabetes before the age of 15 years. The incidence of nephropathy peaks after 10–20 years of type 1 diabetes and declines thereafter, suggesting a possible genetic predisposition to this complication. Although diabetic nephropathy is less common in type 2 diabetes, as this type of diabetes is much more prevalent, most patients with diabetes-related chronic kidney disease will have type 2 diabetes. An increase in patients with end-stage renal disease from type 2 diabetes has been observed even in countries with a low incidence of type 2 diabetes.

Established diabetic nephropathy is preceded by several years of incipient nephropathy, which is characterized by increasing microalbuminuria (albumin excretion rates of 30–300 mg/day), not detectable on dipstick testing. The cumulative incidence of microalbuminuria in patients with type 1 diabetes was 12.6% over 7.3 years in the European Diabetes (EURODIAB) Prospective Complications Study Group. Diabetic nephropathy is more prevalent in certain racial groups such as African Americans and Asians than it is in the white population.

Early detection of microalbuminuria allows intervention to slow the rate of development of diabetic nephropathy (see the following pages).

All patients should be screened for diabetic nephropathy according to agreed protocols (Table 9.6).

The key histological features of diabetic nephropathy are glomerular sclerosis, with thickening of the glomerular basement membrane and mesangial expansion (Figure 9.11).

The cause of diabetic nephropathy is not known, but factors that may be implicated include hyperglycemia-induced hyperfiltration and renal injury, accumulation of advanced glycation endproducts and activation of harmful cytokines.

Patients who have diabetic nephropathy usually exhibit evidence of retinopathy and neuropathy. An absence of retinopathy should suggest the diagnostic possibility of non-diabetic glomerulopathy.

TABLE 9.6

Screening for diabetic nephropathy

- Annually, send a first-pass morning urine sample (provided proteinuria and UTI are absent) for laboratory estimation of albumin:creatinine ratio (all patients with diabetes)
- Serum creatinine and GFR should be measured at the same time
- If an abnormal albumin:creatinine ratio is found (> 2.5 mg/mmol for men, > 3.5 mg/mmol for women), repeat the test twice within 3–4 months. Microalbuminuria is confirmed if a further specimen is abnormal
- Exclude renal disease other than diabetic nephropathy when other factors apply (no significant diabetic retinopathy, resistant hypertension, sudden onset of heavy proteinuria, significant hematuria, rapid deterioration in GFR, patient systemically ill)
- Prescribe an ACE inhibitor and titrate to maximum recommended dose if tolerated when microalbuminuria is confirmed (informed discussion necessary in women with the possibility of pregnancy)
- Substitute an angiotensin-II receptor antagonist if ACE inhibitor is not tolerated
- Maintain blood pressure below 130/80 mmHg

ACE, angiotensin-converting enzyme; GFR, glomerular filtration rate; UTI, urinary tract infection.

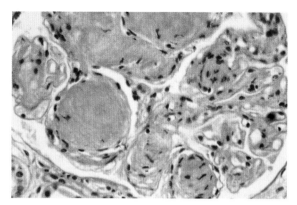

Figure 9.11 Diabetic nephropathy showing diffuse glomerulosclerosis with basement membrane thickening and areas of fibrin deposition called Kimmelstiel–Wilson nodules.

Cerebrovascular disease, carotid artery stenosis, coronary artery disease and peripheral vascular disease are much more common in patients with nephropathy. The hypertension associated with diabetic nephropathy appears to be of renal origin and to occur after the onset of microalbuminuria.

Treatment. Intensive glycemic control has been shown in several studies to slow the progression of diabetic nephropathy. Dietary protein restriction (0.3–0.8 g/kg/day) has also been shown to have a beneficial effect, though is difficult to maintain. In the presence of hypertension, vigorous blood pressure reduction attenuates the decline in renal function and delays progression to end-stage renal failure. A target blood pressure of 120/70 mmHg is usual.

Antihypertensive therapy irrespective of the agent used will slow the development of diabetic nephropathy; however, the use of angiotensin-converting enzyme (ACE) inhibitors to lower blood pressure has been associated with superior clinical benefit in this context, probably because ACE inhibitors reduce intraglomerular capillary pressure, leading to a reduction in proteinuria. Treatment with ACE inhibitors also delays the development of diabetic nephropathy in patients with microalbuminuria. ACE inhibitors have also been demonstrated to have a beneficial effect on diabetic retinopathy. Superiority over conventional agents has also been proven for angiotensin-II receptor antagonists ('blockers', AR2Bs).

Patients with end-stage renal failure resulting from diabetic nephropathy should be offered dialysis and transplantation (as is the case for those without diabetes). Early referral to a nephrologist is recommended and is certainly necessary before serum creatinine reaches 300 µmol/L. Close liaison between the diabetologist and nephrologist to agree when to refer to renal services is best practice. Dialysis may need to be started at a higher glomerular filtration rate than for non-diabetic patients because of a tendency for increased fluid retention and volume-dependent hypertension. The prognosis of diabetic patients receiving hemodialysis and continuous ambulatory dialysis has improved greatly in recent years, but it is still worse than for non-diabetic patients.

Renal transplantation is offered to younger patients, usually with type 1 diabetes, who are free of significant vascular pathology – survival rates are good. Selected patients can be considered for a simultaneous pancreatic transplant (see page 49), particularly those who have had major problems with glycemic control.

The diabetic foot

The development of a foot ulcer is a very dangerous complication of diabetes. Unfortunately, foot ulceration occurs relatively commonly in people with diabetes. Around 15% of patients with diabetes will develop a foot ulcer, and this has enormous associated healthcare costs. Up to 25% of all diabetic hospital admissions in the USA and UK are attributable to foot ulcers. Foot ulceration is a major risk factor for amputations of lower-limb extremities. Adherence to preventive protocols for diabetic footcare can prevent this dire complication of diabetes of which patients know and fear greatly (Table 9.7).

Ulceration of the foot in diabetes almost always occurs on a background of diabetic neuropathy and medium- and small-vessel disease compounded often by abnormal foot biomechanics (Figure 9.12). Loss of pain sensation in the foot allows repeated minor

TABLE 9.7

Footcare advice for patients with diabetic neuropathy

- Keep feet clean; wash in warm water (not hot)
- Use simple emollients to prevent and treat dry cracked skin
- Seek regular foot-care advice from a podiatrist
- Do not wear ill-fitting shoes
- Attend regular feet examinations at the primary care center or hospital clinic
- Report foot problems immediately to podiatrist, nurse or doctor
- Do not self-treat foot problems
- Do not walk barefoot
- Avoid foot contact with hot surfaces
- Ensure there are no objects in shoes before wearing

trauma to go unrecognized by the patient until ulceration has ensued (Figure 9.13). Holidays can be a particularly dangerous time for those with neuropathy because of the risk of injury from walking barefoot, particularly on hot beaches, and the problems caused by wearing ill-fitting sandals. Minor trauma may also precipitate a cascade of events leading to the formation of Charçot arthropathy.

Acute Charçot arthropathy presents with unilateral swelling of the foot with signs of local inflammation (increased skin temperature), erythema and effusion. Pain may occur in more than 75% of patients, although it is often milder than might be expected from the clinical findings. Charçot arthropathy leads to disorganization of the bony architecture of the foot with joint dislocation, fracture and deformity. Deformity of the foot creates areas of high pressure that predispose to callus formation and frank ulceration. Approximately 40% of patients with Charçot arthropathy have concomitant foot ulceration. The presence of callus is, in itself, a predictor of subsequent foot ulceration.

Ulceration of the foot leads to superimposed bacterial infection with organisms such as *Staphylococcus aureus* and *Streptococcus*

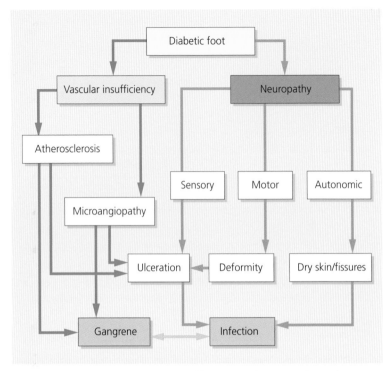

Figure 9.12 Interplay of vascular insufficiency and neuropathy in the development of infection and gangrene in the diabetic foot.

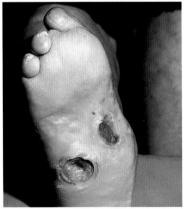

Figure 9.13 Loss of pain sensation due to peripheral neuropathy can lead to prolonged injury to the foot and consequent ulceration. Note the loss of two toes through previous amputation.

pyogenes, often accompanied by anaerobes such as *Bacteroides* spp. Infected diabetic foot ulcers exhibit signs of inflammation – erythema, warmth and tenderness – though such signs may be relatively mild despite significant underlying infection. Serious complications such as deep-seated infection and osteomyelitis may occur. Diagnosing underlying osteomyelitis can prove difficult. MRI is a helpful diagnostic tool. Early recognition of this serious complication of diabetic foot ulceration is necessary so that prompt treatment can be instigated. Ischemic ulcers can also occur in diabetic patients, but with a much lower frequency than neuropathic ulcers.

Treatment of diabetic foot ulcers lacks an evidence base. It requires substantial expertise and considerable experience. A multidisciplinary approach should lead to the involvement of diabetologists, podiatrists, vascular surgeons, orthopedic surgeons, microbiologists, primary care providers, nurses and orthotists. Adequate debridement of slough and necrotic tissue combined with antibiotic treatment of infected lesions form the first principles of therapy. Pressure relief using insoles or casts, such as a total-contact cast or the Scotchcast boot, promotes ulcer healing. Despite these interventions, many patients require surgery. More than 60% of non-traumatic lower-limb amputations occur in people with diabetes. Novel therapies, such as the use of bioengineered skin substitutes, have been developed but none is backed by sufficient evidence to become an accepted part of the standard treatment of foot ulcers.

Hypertension and major vascular disease

In the WHO Multinational Study of Vascular Disease in Diabetes, cardiovascular disease was the most common cause of death, accounting for 44% of deaths in type 1 diabetes and 52% of deaths in type 2 diabetes. Diabetes is associated with a two- to fourfold increase in the risk of coronary artery disease, cerebrovascular disease and peripheral-limb ischemia (Figure 9.14). Diabetic patients, particularly women, have an increased risk of dying from coronary artery disease and an increased mortality from peripheral vascular disease. Of all lower-limb amputations, 50% are performed on diabetic patients. Atherosclerosis is more severe and widespread in diabetic patients, and consequently coronary artery disease may present at a younger age

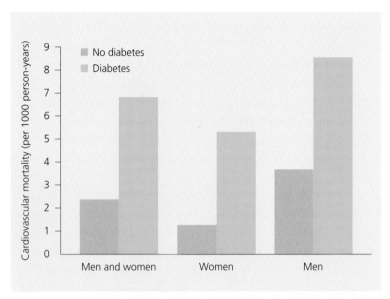

Figure 9.14 Mortality from cardiovascular disease is higher in diabetic patients than in non-diabetic individuals. Data were collected from 1976 to 2001 and are from Preis et al. 2009. Note that the risk increases further when major risk factors (hypercholesterolemia, diastolic hypertension and smoking) are present.

than in the non-diabetic population. Diabetic patients have more multivessel disease of the coronary arteries. They also have an increase in left ventricular mass. While this may be partly related to the increased prevalence of hypertension in this population, diabetes appears to be an independent contributor to left ventricular mass. This fact and other considerable pathological, epidemiological and clinical data point to the existence of a specific diabetic cardiomyopathy.

Risk factors for macrovascular disease in diabetic patients include those that apply to the background population, but hypertension and hyperlipidemia are particularly important in patients with type 2 diabetes. Hemostatic abnormalities such as decreased fibrinolysis and increased fibrinogen levels are also relevant, as are elevated levels of plasminogen activator inhibitor type 1 and the putative relationship between hyperinsulinemia and atherosclerosis.

While lipid levels in type 1 diabetes reflect those in the background population, patients with type 2 diabetes typically have an abnormal lipid profile referred to as diabetic dyslipidemia, with raised triglyceride levels and low levels of HDL cholesterol. Vigorous treatment of hyperlipidemia is a standard aspect of diabetes management to reduce death and morbidity from premature vascular disease.

The detection and treatment of hypertension is a vital part of overall diabetes care. Hypertension is common in people with diabetes, affecting 10–30% of white patients with type 1 diabetes and 30–50% of patients with type 2 diabetes. In NHANES III, 71% of diabetic patients were found to have hypertension. The emergence of hypertension in type 1 diabetes may reflect the onset of diabetic nephropathy. Hypertension in diabetes substantially increases the risk of both microvascular and macrovascular disease.

In the UK Prospective Diabetes Study (UKPDS), each 10 mmHg decrease in mean systolic pressure was associated with a reduction in risk of 12% for any complication related to diabetes, 15% for risk of death related to diabetes, 11% for risk of myocardial infarction and 13% for risk of microvascular complications. In the Heart Outcomes Prevention Evaluation (HOPE) study, ramipril reduced the rates of death, myocardial infarction and stroke in a broad range of high-risk patients, 40% of whom had diabetes. In the Hypertension Optimal Treatment (HOT) study, intensive treatment of blood pressure to achieve a target of 140/81 mmHg was associated with a 66% reduction in mortality in people with diabetes. Multiple drug therapy was necessary to achieve this target. This study also showed that in people with diabetes, blood pressure needed to be lowered further than in those without diabetes to achieve equivalent benefit on mortality. Table 9.8 shows the risk reductions for macro- and microvascular outcomes associated with intensive blood pressure reduction in the UKPDS.

Epidemiological evidence indicates the benefit of reducing systolic blood pressure to below 130 mmHg, and a treatment goal of blood pressure below 130/80 mmHg is widely accepted for patients with diabetes (even lower in patients with diabetic nephropathy).

TABLE 9.8

The effect of intensive blood pressure reduction on microvascular and macrovascular outcomes in patients with type 2 diabetes in the 10-year UKPDS

Outcome	Risk reduction (%)
Diabetes-related endpoints	24
Deaths related to diabetes	32
Stroke	44
Microvascular endpoints	37

UKPDS, UK Prospective Diabetes Study.

A number of studies have demonstrated that ACE inhibitors reduce urinary albumin excretion rates, delay the development of proteinuria in those with microalbuminuria and reduce the risk of dialysis, renal transplantation and death; these findings make ACE inhibitors the drugs of first choice in the treatment of hypertension in diabetic patients. ACE inhibitors are also effective in decreasing cardiovascular morbidity and mortality in patients with congestive cardiac failure and in those who have had a myocardial infarction. AR2Bs have a renoprotective effect similar to ACE inhibitors. Most hypertensive diabetic patients will require multiple drug therapy to reach the recommended targets outlined above. Additional drugs useful as add-on therapy are β-blockers, low-dose thiazide diuretics, calcium antagonists and α-blockers. However, in many studies, the use of a thiazide diuretic or a β-blocker has been associated with an increased likelihood of developing diabetes that is not seen with ACE inhibitors. Indeed, there has been a suggestion that the use of ACE inhibitors may actually protect from the development of diabetes. As a result of the possibility of increased risk of diabetes when using a thiazide diuretic, it is best to use the lowest effective dose.

Erectile dysfunction

Failure of erection is a common complication of diabetes in men (see *Fast Facts: Erectile Dysfunction*). It occurs with an estimated prevalence of 38–55%. Erectile dysfunction is now viewed, in most cases, as a vascular complication of diabetes. It is most likely to result from a defect in nitric-oxide-mediated smooth-muscle relaxation as a consequence of autonomic nerve damage and endothelial dysfunction. Large-vessel disease may also play a role.

Treatment. Erectile dysfunction in diabetes responds to the use of phosphodiesterase inhibitors such as sildenafil, vardenafil and tadalafil. The success rate for sildenafil in the treatment of diabetic erectile dysfunction is in the order of 60%.

Alternative strategies when phosphodiesterase inhibitors fail include intracavernosal injection of alprostadil (prostaglandin E) and the transurethral insertion of a pellet containing alprostadil and polyethylene glycol; discontinuation rates are high, however.

Passive penile tumescence to allow intercourse may be achieved by applying a vacuum to the penis using a hand- or battery-operated pump, with penile engorgement being maintained using a rubber constrictive ring at the base of the penis. Surgical implantation of a penile prosthesis can be successful in carefully selected cases.

Other diabetic complications

Diabetes mellitus is associated with many other manifestations, some relatively common, others rather rare.

Non-alcoholic fatty liver disease. There is a growing recognition of non-alcoholic fatty liver disease (NAFLD) as a complication of diabetes, and indeed this condition may even be a precursor of type 2 diabetes. NAFLD takes many forms, from the relatively mild simple steatosis through non-alcoholic steatohepatitis to advanced fibrosis and cirrhosis.

Skin conditions. Many skin conditions are associated with diabetes; these include necrobiosis lipoidica diabeticorum, diabetic dermopathy and diabetic bullae. Diabetic cheiroarthropathy occurs as limited joint mobility with thickening and tightening of the skin, and is most commonly seen in the hands (the 'prayer' sign). Dupuytren's contracture and adhesive capsulitis are frequently encountered in diabetic patients, though there may be no specific link to diabetes.

Mental health considerations

Individuals with diabetes often have to make major lifestyle changes, which in the longer term can affect mental health. Changes to food intake and physical activity (see Chapter 8), the constant pressures of weight management (sometimes exacerbated by diabetes medications that cause weight gain), and the prospect of regular painful insulin injections and blood glucose checks can become overwhelming. In addition to the risk of complications and comorbidities already discussed in this chapter, diabetes can also affect general health (for example, the severe fatigue and somnolence associated with poorly controlled diabetes). It is understandable that all of these factors, either individually or together, can cause distress and dysphoria, and contribute to low mood. It is therefore important to recognize psychological stress and depression in people with diabetes, and to consider how as healthcare professionals we may offer support.

Depression. Diabetes is associated with high rates (up to 60% in some series) of depressive symptoms. Depression is also a risk factor for diabetes, since depression is associated with an increase in sedentary lifestyle, poor diet and weight gain; some antidepressants also promote weight gain. Whilst it is simple to state that diabetes causes depression, or depression causes diabetes, there is also evidence to suggest that diabetes and depression may develop in parallel and may have common biological etiologies.

Other mental illnesses. Diabetes also occurs at a more frequent rate in people with mental illnesses such as schizophrenia and bipolar disease. Antipsychotics can cause major weight gain and an increase in sedentary lifestyle, thus promoting insulin resistance and increased diabetes risk. However, older data show that before the availability of antipsychotic medication, people with schizophrenia had unexpectedly higher rates of diabetes. This indicates that psychotic illnesses increase diabetes susceptibility, an association that is now worsened by the weight-promoting effects of the antipsychotic drugs used.

Strategies to prevent weight gain in people with major mental illness include lifestyle interventions, such as supported eating and exercise regimens, when antipsychotic drugs are initiated. Short-term studies also show that metformin can be of benefit.

Strategies to improve adherence to recommendations

Inflexible clinical recommendations applied without engagement with the person with diabetes does not engender a working partnership between patient and healthcare professional that will meet our common goals: good health for the long term. Inflexibility also leads to rebellious behaviors by patients, often to their metabolic detriment.

It is therefore important to develop an open dialogue with patients and to enquire into factors that may be undermining their self care. Look for external factors such as long working hours or travel times, which may limit opportunities for physical activity or cooking of healthy meals. Are there underlying stresses, such as interpersonal tensions with partners or other family members? Is someone undermining the efforts made at lifestyle change? Is there underlying depression that requires intervention?

Numerous factors can affect glucose control, including medication failure, stresses or frustrations at work or home, or the loss of a pet, despite the patient's rigorous adherence to lifestyle and drug regimens. This can be emotionally distressing, as the individual's efforts are not repaid by good control or health professional praise, and can lead to an 'I may as well throw in the towel' mentality and periods of even poorer control.

The detrimental impact of these events can be avoided by early active intervention by healthcare professionals to identify the cause of poor glucose control and remedy it. Patients should also be encouraged to see the same healthcare professional, since developing a supportive (but not dependent) therapeutic relationship for the longer term helps detect 'treatment fatigue' early.

Consulting a psychologist may be useful, since a number of interventions may assist with depression and adherence issues. People with major mental illness may require review by their general practitioner or a psychiatrist for further management.

For information technology (IT)-savvy people, there are now a number of programs that can link between glucose monitors and computer devices. These programs can help patients and their clinicians examine patterns in blood glucose levels. However, these types of devices should be used with caution, as in some instances an excess of data can become overwhelming and may even add to the burden of self-care.

Key points – complications and mental health considerations

- Chronic complications of diabetes may be microvascular or macrovascular.
- Many different types of neuropathy affect diabetic patients, with some being very debilitating.
- All diabetic patients must be screened for the presence of retinopathy and referred for ophthalmic review where necessary.
- Diabetic nephropathy is the leading cause of chronic renal failure in western societies.
- Treatment of diabetic nephropathy with blood-pressure reduction and angiotensin-converting enzyme (ACE) inhibitors slows disease progression.
- Neuropathy and ischemia increase the risk of foot ulceration, which is associated with enormous healthcare costs.
- Major vascular disease accounts for more than half of all deaths in diabetes.
- Lowering of blood pressure to 130/80 mmHg is associated with a considerable reduction in vascular morbidity and microvascular disease.
- Failure of erection occurs in 38–55% of men with diabetes.
- It is important to recognize psychological stress and depression in patients with diabetes, as lifestyle changes associated with the condition can be overwhelming for some.
- Open dialogue between healthcare professional and patient is important in order to identify factors that may be undermining self care, and to rectify poor glucose control early.

Key references

Boulton AJM, Vileikyte L, Ragnarson-Tennvall G, Apelqvist J. The global burden of diabetic foot disease. *Lancet* 2005;366:1719–24. (The issue also contains other relevant articles on diabetic foot disease.)

Bril V, England J, Franklin GM et al. Evidence-based guideline: Treatment of painful diabetic neuropathy: report of the American Academy of Neurology, the American Association of Neuromuscular and Electrodiagnostic Medicine, and the American Academy of Physical Medicine and Rehabilitation. *Neurology* 2011;76:1758–65.

de Boer IH, Rue TC, Hall YN et al. Temporal trends in the prevalence of diabetic kidney disease in the United States. *JAMA* 2011;305:2532–9.

Fong DS, Aiello L, Gardner TW et al. Diabetic retinopathy. *Diabetes Care* 2003;26:S99–102.

Heart Outcomes Prevention Evaluation (HOPE) Study Investigators. Effects of ramipril on cardiovascular and microvascular outcomes in people with diabetes mellitus: results of the HOPE study and MICRO-HOPE substudy. *Lancet* 2000;355:253–9.

Klein R, Klein BE, Moss SE. Visual impairment in diabetes. *Ophthalmology* 1984;91:1–9.

Lewis EJ, Hunsicker LG, Bain RP, Rohde BS. The effect of angiotensin-converting-enzyme inhibition on diabetic nephropathy. *N Engl J Med* 1993;329:1456–62.

Morrish NJ, Wang SL, Stevens LK et al. Mortality and causes of death in the WHO Multinational Study of Vascular Disease in Diabetes. *Diabetologia* 2001;44(suppl 2):S14–21.

Preis SR, Hwang SJ, Coady S et al. Trends in all-cause and cardiovascular disease mortality among women and men with and without diabetes mellitus in the Framingham Heart Study, 1950 to 2005. *Circulation* 2009;119:1728–35.

UK Prospective Diabetes Study Group. Tight blood pressure control and risk of macrovascular and microvascular complications in type 2 diabetes: UKPDS 38. *BMJ* 1998;317:703–13.

Vinik AL, Park TS, Stansberry KB, Pittenger GL. Diabetic neuropathies. *Diabetologia* 2000;43:957–73.

Vinik A, Richardson D. Erectile dysfunction in diabetes. *Clinical Diabetes* 1996;14:111–20.

Watkins PJ. The diabetic foot. *BMJ* 2003;326:977–9.

Ziegler D. Painful diabetic neuropathy: treatment and future aspects. *Diabetes Metab Res Rev* 2008;24:S52–7.

Acute hypoglycemia potentially threatens the quality of life on a daily basis for people with type 1 diabetes. It may also affect patients with type 2 diabetes, especially those who are treated with sulfonylureas or insulin. Hypoglycemia represents a considerable barrier to the goal of achievement of near-normal blood glucose levels in insulin-treated patients. It is feared by patients with diabetes treated with insulin and has the capacity to seriously disrupt their lives.

Symptoms

The symptoms of hypoglycemia are listed in Table 10.1. The initial symptoms of hypoglycemia are caused by sympathoadrenal activation. Such symptoms include sweating, shakiness, palpitation, anxiety and a sensation of hunger. Patients come to recognize their own hypoglycemic symptoms, which are often highly individualized. If hypoglycemia is not reversed promptly then patients may go on to develop symptoms due to neuroglycopenia (resulting from brain neuronal glucose deprivation) and these symptoms include behavioral changes, cognitive dysfunction and even seizures and coma.

Less commonly, some patients may not experience initial sympathetic symptoms and present with neuroglycopenia, a complication known as hypoglycemic unawareness. Hypoglycemia

TABLE 10.1

Symptoms of hypoglycemia

- Hunger
- Anxiety
- Tremor
- Sweating
- Palpitation
- Lightheadedness/dizziness
- Tiredness
- Difficulty concentrating or thinking logically
- Confusion

unawareness is a potentially reversible situation with expert help. In people with type 1 diabetes, 2–4% of deaths have been attributed to hypoglycemia.

People with type 1 diabetes experience symptomatic hypoglycemia on average twice per week, with significant disabling hypoglycemia occurring approximately once a year. Hypoglycemia is much less common in people with type 2 diabetes but frequently goes unrecognized. In the UK Hypoglycaemia Study Group, there was a low incidence of hypoglycemia in those taking oral hypoglycemic drugs, but an appreciable incidence in those on insulin therapy. The glucose threshold that triggers hypoglycemia in diabetic patients is different from that in people without diabetes. Hypoglycemia may be experienced at a higher plasma glucose threshold in patients with poorly controlled diabetes, while patients with tightly controlled diabetes may tolerate remarkably low plasma glucose levels without experiencing hypoglycemic symptoms.

Unawareness

It is generally recommended that patients avoid having glucose concentrations below 4 mmol/L (72 mg/dL), as frequent exposure to glucose levels below this threshold may result in the aforementioned phenomenon of hypoglycemic unawareness. Lack of awareness of hypoglycemia poses a hazardous situation for those who are driving or exposed to heavy machinery or other dangers.

Causes

Hypoglycemia in diabetes is a consequence of absolute or relative excess of exogenously administered insulin or endogenous insulin secretion. The causes are shown in Table 10.2.

Death

Death from hypoglycemia is rare, but it may follow excess alcohol consumption or deliberate insulin overdose. Occasionally, tragically unexpected deaths happen in young patients with type 1 diabetes; these often occur in bed and it has been speculated that they may result from hypoglycemia-induced cardiac dysrhythmias.

TABLE 10.2

Causes of hypoglycemia

- Excess or ill-timed insulin dose
- Deficient glucose delivery
  - missed meals or snacks
  - overnight fasting
  - effect of alcohol (suppression of hepatic glucose output)
- Increased use of glucose during exercise
- Reduced clearance of insulin in renal failure
- Increased insulin sensitivity causing late hypoglycemia (e.g. after prolonged exercise)

Treatment

Most episodes of hypoglycemia are self-treated and respond quickly to the ingestion of glucose tablets, fruit juices or a soft drink. As hypoglycemia may recur promptly, individuals are recommended to have a snack or meal once the initial hypoglycemia is corrected. When hypoglycemia is so severe that the patient is unwilling or unable to take anything orally, parenteral therapy is required.

Partners, parents, relatives or close associates of people with type 1 diabetes should be taught how to inject the affected individual with glucagon, 1 mg intramuscularly or subcutaneously (followed by the ingestion of carbohydrates to restore hepatic glycogen). If this is not effective within 10 minutes, medical staff should administer 50 mL of 20% glucose by intravenous infusion into a large vein through a large-gauge needle. If 10% glucose is used, a larger volume will be required to correct the hypoglycemia. A 50% glucose solution is not recommended because of irritant damage to veins.

Follow-up

In all instances it is important that efforts be made to identify the cause of hypoglycemia, particularly when it is recurrent or unrecognized by the individual, and to formulate a suitable course of action to prevent future hypoglycemic events.

Key points – hypoglycemia

- Symptomatic hypoglycemia is common in patients with type 1 diabetes.
- Hypoglycemia is a barrier to the achievement of tight glycemic control.
- Frequent hypoglycemia may lead to the development of hypoglycemia unawareness.
- There are many and varied causes of hypoglycemia.
- Death from hypoglycemia is rare.

Key references

Cranston I, Lomas J, Maran A et al. Restoration of hypoglycaemia awareness in patients with long-duration insulin-dependent diabetes. *Lancet* 1994;344:283–7.

Cryer PE. *Hypoglycemia: Pathophysiology, Diagnosis and Treatment.* New York: Oxford University Press, 1997.

Cryer PE, Davis SN, Shamoon H. Hypoglycemia in Diabetes. *Diabetes Care* 2003;26:1902–12.

Fanelli CG, Porcellati F, Pampanelli S, Bolli GB. Insulin therapy and hypoglycaemia: the size of the problem. *Diabet Metab Res Rev* 2004;20(suppl 2);S32–42.

Fisher M. Hypoglycaemia in patients with type 2 diabetes: minimising the risk. *Br J Diabetes Vasc Dis* 2010;10:35–41.

Frier BM. How hypoglycaemia can affect the life of a person with diabetes. *Diabet Metab Res Rev* 2008;24:247–52.

McAuley V, Deary IJ, Frier BM. Symptoms of hypoglycaemia in people with diabetes. *Diabet Med* 2001;18:690–705.

Diabetic ketoacidosis

Diabetic ketoacidosis (DKA) is a serious life-threatening complication of type 1 diabetes. DKA occurs more often in adults than in children, but it can occur at any age. Most commonly seen in young adults, it is the main cause of death in type 1 diabetic patients under the age of 20 years.

DKA may also be encountered in people with type 2 diabetes, particularly in those of Afro-Caribbean descent. When DKA occurs in type 2 diabetes, it is the physiological stress caused by the underlying illness that precipitates the acute metabolic decompensation.

Definition. DKA consists of the biochemical triad of ketonemia, hyperglycemia and acidemia. Biochemically, it is defined as an increase in the concentrations of ketones (3-hydroxybutyrate) of 3 mmol/L (> 31.2 mg/dL) or over (or significant ketonuria of more than 2+ on standard urine ketone sticks), blood glucose over 11 mmol/L (198 mg/dL) or known diabetes and serum bicarbonate below 15 mmol/L (15 mEq/L) and/or venous pH below 7.3.

Causes. DKA may occasionally be the presenting manifestation of type 1 diabetes or, more often in patients with established diabetes, it is the consequence of many precipitating factors, of which the most common is infection (accounting for 30–50% of cases; Table 11.1).

Of the infective causes, urinary tract infection and pneumonia predominate. Other common medical conditions such as myocardial infarction, acute stroke, pancreatitis and trauma may precipitate DKA. Alcohol or drug abuse may also contribute. Newly diagnosed, previously unknown type 1 diabetes causes about 15% of cases. Missed insulin injections account for about 25% of cases. Often, psychological factors are implicated if there has been deliberate insulin omission or non-compliance with insulin therapeutic regimens.

TABLE 11.1

Precipitating causes of diabetic ketoacidosis

- Infection (e.g. urinary tract, pneumonia, viral)
- Acute medical illness (e.g. myocardial infarction, stroke)
- Acute surgical illness (e.g. pancreatitis, appendicitis)
- Trauma
- Insulin omission
- Inappropriate reduction in insulin dose
- Psychological factors
- Alcohol or drug abuse
- Eating disorders
- Unidentified

Frequent recurrent DKA in one individual is a commonly encountered clinical scenario – it is usually the consequence of a psychosocial problem that may be very difficult to delineate. The incidence of DKA is slightly greater in females than in males. Recurrent DKA in young women is frequently caused by insulin omission. Eating disorders can be an important contributory factor. However, no definite cause is found in a large proportion of cases of DKA.

Clinical presentation. DKA is characterized by hyperglycemia, hyperketonemia and metabolic acidosis, which occur as a consequence of insulin deficiency or ineffectiveness, accompanied by increased circulating concentrations of counter-regulatory hormones (cortisol, growth hormone, glucagon and catecholamines) (Figure 11.1).

Hyperglycemia results principally from increased hepatic glucose production with a contribution from increased renal glucose production and decreased glucose uptake into peripheral tissues. Increased lipolysis leads to a massive rise in ketone bodies (acetone, β-hydroxybutyrate and acetoacetate); as these are strong organic acids, this produces a metabolic acidosis and the rapid increase in hydrogen ions exceeds the buffering capacity of the kidneys. Hyperglycemia and

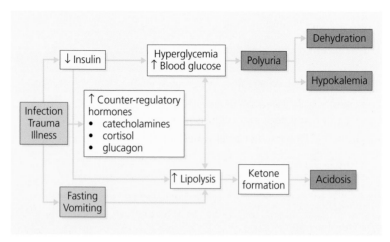

Figure 11.1 The pathogenesis of diabetic ketoacidosis.

hyperketonemia cause an osmotic diuresis leading to hypovolemia, dehydration and loss of electrolytes – notably sodium and potassium.

Symptoms of DKA develop rapidly, usually within 24 hours, and consist of nausea and vomiting (induced by ketones and contributing to fluid and electrolyte disturbance), thirst and polyuria (Table 11.2). Abdominal pain is common, occurring in 40–75% of cases and occasionally mimicking an acute abdomen. Failure to recognize this, particularly if operative intervention is undertaken, may have fatal

TABLE 11.2

Symptoms of diabetic ketoacidosis

- Nausea
- Vomiting
- Thirst
- Polyuria
- Abdominal pain
- Dyspnea
- Confusion
- Symptoms of precipitating illness

consequences, though the possibility of an acute abdomen should not be overlooked.

In addition to the physical signs that may reflect the underlying condition causing DKA, there will be signs of dehydration including tachycardia and hypotension. Acetone may be smelled on the breath as a fruity odor and acidosis may result in labored Kussmaul respiration. The conscious level varies between normality and mild alteration of consciousness: coma is relatively rare.

Biochemical tests will confirm the diagnosis of DKA (hyperglycemia, ketonemia, ketonuria and acidosis). In addition to plasma glucose and arterial blood gas measurements, all patients should have a full blood count, and urea, electrolytes and creatinine should be measured. In all cases the underlying cause of DKA should be sought, with tests that may include, for example, chest radiography, electrocardiography and cultures of blood and urine. Patients with DKA may have leukocytosis in the absence of infection. The initial potassium level may be low, normal or high (most frequently elevated) in the face of a profound potassium deficit. Patients with initial hypokalemia are considered to have severe serious total body potassium depletion. Potassium loss is caused by a shift of potassium from the intracellular to the extracellular space in exchange for hydrogen ions. Much of the shifted extracellular potassium is lost in the urine because of osmotic diuresis (compounded by further loss due to vomiting).

Treatment. Immediate treatment of any identifiable cause of the DKA should be undertaken without delay. Until recently, standard management of DKA focused on reducing blood glucose levels with insulin and intravenous fluids. There is still universal agreement that the initial cornerstone of treatment is fluid replacement and insulin administration. The intravascular volume should be expanded to correct a typical deficit of 100 mL/kg of water with intravenous isotonic saline, which will also improve renal perfusion. Infusion rates of 1 L per hour for the first hour, 1 L for the next 2 hours and 1 L over the next 4 hours are usually adequate except in those patients with profound hypovolemia and hypotension, who may need twice this amount (see Table 11.3). If the initial systolic blood pressure is below 90 mmHg, 500 mL of normal saline should be given over 15 minutes. In the presence of significant hypernatremia, isotonic saline can be replaced with 0.45% saline. The aim is to replace total body deficits of water and electrolytes, with half the estimated deficit being replaced in 12–24 hours (Table 11.3). Once the blood glucose has fallen to about 14 mmol/L (252 mg/dL), saline should be replaced with 5% dextrose (or an infusion of 10% glucose given at 125 mL/hour started alongside the infusion of normal saline to correct circulatory volume) to allow continued insulin administration to suppress ketogenesis while avoiding hypoglycemia.

Insulin is best administered by low-dose continuous intravenous infusion. Formerly insulin was infused at a rate of 5–10 units/hour to produce steady-state insulin levels, to inhibit lipolysis and hence ketogenesis and to inhibit hepatic glucose production and enhance disposal of glucose and ketone bodies by peripheral tissues. The insulin infusion rate can be determined by hourly capillary blood glucose measurements to maintain the blood glucose level between 5 and 10 mmol/L (90 and 180 mg/dL). Modern guidelines have moved towards a treatment strategy that, in addition to replacing fluid and electrolytes, aims to resolve ketonemia, and advocate a policy of measuring blood ketones as an index of treatment success. In parallel

TABLE 11.3

Typical fluid and electrolyte losses in diabetic ketoacidosis

Water	5–10 L
Sodium	400–700 mmol
Chloride	300–600 mmol
Potassium	≥ 300–700 mmol
Magnesium	30–60 mmol
Phosphate	50–100 mmol
Calcium	50–100 mmol
Alkali	300–500 mmol

with this, it is recommended that insulin 'sliding scales' are replaced with a weight-based fixed rate insulin infusion of 0.1 units of insulin/ kg bodyweight. Measurement of venous pH and bicarbonate rather than arterial values is also advised. In the last few years, continuation of subcutaneous long-acting basal analogs has become widespread practice to provide background insulin when the insulin infusion is stopped and prevent rebound hyperglycemia.

Insulin therapy and correction of acidosis decreases potassium levels, and most patients will require intravenous potassium supplementation to prevent hypokalemia and replace total body potassium deficit. The use of bicarbonate to correct acidosis is not recommended as studies have failed to show any benefit from bicarbonate administration, which may actually be harmful.

Once ketoacidosis is resolved, hyperglycemia has been corrected and the patient has improved clinically and is eating and drinking, subcutaneous insulin administration can resume.

Prognosis. The prognosis of DKA is usually determined by the precipitating cause. The overall mortality is 3–4%. Cerebral edema is a rare life-threatening complication usually encountered in children with DKA (around 1% of episodes). It carries a mortality of 40–90% and manifests as a decreasing level of consciousness, with headache, seizures, papilledema, bradycardia and respiratory arrest. Treatment is with intravenous mannitol. Mechanical ventilation may help to reduce swelling of the brain. In the UK, 70–80% of diabetes-related deaths in children under 12 years of age are caused by cerebral edema.

When a patient presents with DKA, every effort should be made to identify the cause where possible in order to establish strategies to prevent a recurrence.

Hyperosmolar hyperglycemic state

Hyperosmolar hyperglycemic state (HHS) is one of the two serious metabolic derangements in diabetes that may be life-threatening. It is less common than DKA, but carries a higher mortality rate (10–20%). Other terms used to describe the condition include diabetic hyperosmolar non-ketoacidotic coma, hyperosmolar hyperglycemic non-ketotic coma and hyperosmolar non-ketotic state. HHS is characterized by severe hyperglycemia, dehydration and hyperosmolarity in the absence of ketonemia/ketonuria and acidosis (Table 11.4).

HHS usually occurs in middle-aged or elderly patients with type 2 diabetes (often undiagnosed). The absence of ketoacidosis in HHS is not fully explained but may be because such individuals have insulin levels low enough to cause hyperglycemia but adequate to inhibit lipolysis and ketogenesis because of the differential effect of insulin on lipolysis and glucose uptake. HHS occurs in patients with type 2 diabetes in the presence of a concomitant illness that leads to reduced fluid intake. Infection (commonly urinary tract infection and pneumonia) is the preceding illness in 30–60% of cases. Other relatively frequent causes include myocardial infarction, stroke and concomitant drug use such as thiazide diuretics or corticosteroids.

Clinical presentation. Typically, patients have symptoms of diabetes and weakness. A wide variety of focal neurological abnormalities (for example, focal or generalized seizures, hemiparesis) or global neurologic abnormalities (for example, drowsiness, delirium, coma) may be present. Patients are clinically severely volume-depleted and often there are signs of infection when this is the precipitating cause.

Treatment of HHS by fluid, electrolyte and insulin replacement is as for DKA (fluid deficits may be large [for example, 10 L or more]). Attention should be focused on the underlying cause when identifiable.

TABLE 11.4

Clinical features of hyperosmolar hyperglycemic state

- Severe hyperglycemia: plasma glucose > 50 mmol/L (900 mg/dL)
- Severe dehydration and hyperosmolality > 340 mOsm/kg
- No hyperketonemia and no acidosis: bicarbonate > 18 mmol/L (18 mEq/L)
- Precipitating factors (e.g. diuretic use, ingestion of high-glucose drinks, infection, renal impairment)

Thromboembolic events occur in HHS and treatment with low-molecular-weight heparin is recommended for those with established thromboembolic disease, immobility or risk factors for venous thrombosis.

Key points – diabetic ketoacidosis and hyperosmolar hyperglycemic state

- Diabetic ketoacidosis (DKA) is a life-threatening complication of type 1 diabetes.
- DKA is characterized by hyperglycemia, hyperketonemia and acidosis.
- Infection is the most common precipitating factor in DKA.
- Treatment of DKA is by fluid and electrolyte replacement, intravenous insulin and treatment of the underlying cause, when known.
- The overall mortality of DKA is 3–4%.
- Hyperosmolar hyperglycemic state (HHS) occurs in older patients with type 2 diabetes.
- HHS is similar to DKA, but without ketosis and acidosis.
- Treatment of HHS is similar to the treatment of DKA.

Key references

Campbell IW, Duncan LJ, Innes JA et al. Abdominal pain in diabetic metabolic decompensation: clinical significance. *JAMA* 1975;233:166–8.

Kitabchi AE, Umpierrez GE, Miles JM, Fisher JN. Hyperglycemic crises in adult patients with diabetes. *Diabetes Care* 2009;32:1335–43.

Morris LR, Murphy MB, Kitabchi AE. Bicarbonate therapy in severe diabetic ketoacidosis. *Ann Intern Med* 1986;105:836–40.

Polonsky WH, Anderson BJ, Lohrer PA et al. Insulin omission in women with IDDM. *Diabetes Care* 1994;17:1178–85.

Silver SM, Clark EC, Schroeder BM, Sterns RH. Pathogenesis of cerebral edema after treatment of diabetic ketoacidosis. *Kidney Int* 1997;51:1237–44.

Umperriez GE, Murphy MB, Kitabchi AE. Diabetic ketoacidosis and hyperglycemic hyperosmolar syndrome. *Diabetes Spectrum* 2002;15:28–36.

White NH. Diabetic ketoacidosis in children. *Endocrinol Metab Clin North Am* 2000;29:657–82.

Diabetic pregnancy is associated with an increased risk of adverse outcome for the fetus, but there is little excess mortality among diabetic women. Pregnancy may be complicated by type 1 diabetes, gestational diabetes mellitus (GDM) and, increasingly, by type 2 diabetes. Occasionally, both types 1 and 2 may be diagnosed for the first time during pregnancy. Of all pregnancies in the USA, 3–10% are complicated by diabetes (90% are cases of GDM). Prevalence is higher in certain ethnic groups such as Asian, Afro-Caribbean and Hispanic groups. The fetal morbidity associated with diabetes is shown in Table 12.1.

There is a miscarriage rate of 9–14% among women with pre-existing diabetes. Higher rates are seen in those with very poor glycemic control. The risk of a structural anomaly in the fetus is four to eight times the rate in the normal population. The congenital malformation rate in diabetic pregnancy is 5.1–9.8%. Two-thirds of the birth defects affect the cardiovascular and central nervous systems, with neural tube defects being particularly common. The achievement of meticulous preconception glycemic control can reduce the incidence of malformation to near normal.

TABLE 12.1

Fetal morbidity in diabetic pregnancy

• Miscarriage	• Birth injury
• Birth defects	• Polycythemia
• Growth restriction	• Neonatal hypoglycemia
• Growth acceleration	• Neonatal hypocalcemia
• Fetal obesity	• Postnatal hyperbilirubinemia
• Increased perinatal mortality	• Fetal respiratory distress syndrome

Diabetic pregnancy is linked with the development of large-for-gestational-age babies, but growth restriction in patients with pre-existing type 1 diabetes may also occur, particularly when the diabetes is associated with vascular complications. Fetal macrosomia (affecting 15–45% of babies born to diabetic women) is a frequent complication of diabetic pregnancy and increases the likelihood of birth injuries such as shoulder dystocia and brachial plexus trauma. Perinatal mortality has fallen greatly in diabetic pregnancies but remains approximately twice that observed in non-diabetic pregnancies, with serious congenital malformations accounting for a large proportion of fetal loss.

Management of a diabetic pregnancy

Preconception. The management of existing diabetes must start in the preconception period. Preparation for conception must be discussed with women of childbearing age. The insulin regimen should be optimized to achieve a glycated hemoglobin (HbA_{1c}) below 6.5% (48 mmol/mol) without unacceptable hypoglycemia, although in practice this often proves difficult to achieve. Women should take folic acid, 5 mg daily, to reduce the risk of neural tube defects.

After conception women should be seen as soon as possible in a combined diabetic/obstetric clinic with access to a dedicated diabetes physician, obstetrician, diabetes specialist nurse, dietitian and midwife. Blood glucose levels should be checked in the fasting state and 1 hour after each meal. Frequent visits are necessary to achieve target blood glucose values of 5.0–5.5 mmol/L (90–99 mg/dL) fasting and below 7.8 mmol/L (140 mg/dL) postprandially (fasting glucose targets recommended by the UK National Institute for Health and Clinical Excellence are 3.5–5.9 mmol/L [63–106 mg/dL]). Dietary therapy should avoid single large meals and meals/food with a large percentage of simple carbohydrates.

Metformin can be continued throughout the pregnancy by a woman with type 2 diabetes, though most women will require additional insulin. Women with type 1 diabetes should be advised of an increased risk of hypoglycemia and hypoglycemic unawareness in the first trimester. The effectiveness of continuous subcutaneous insulin infusion (insulin pump therapy), particularly for those women who cannot achieve acceptable glucose control or experience troublesome hypoglycemia, is well established.

Cardiac anomaly scans should be offered at 20 weeks' gestation and scans to assess fetal growth and amniotic fluid volume at 28 weeks, 32 weeks and 36 weeks. Planning of the optimal timing and mode of delivery should be made prospectively.

Insulin-treated women are best managed by an insulin pump regimen during labor or Cesarean section.

Effect on complications. Pregnancy may be hazardous to women with pre-existing complications of diabetes. Diabetic retinopathy may deteriorate and women with diabetic nephropathy may experience a decline in renal function and an increase in proteinuria. A successful outcome of pregnancy is unlikely when the serum creatinine exceeds 250 µmol/L. Close monitoring is mandatory, with retinal assessment at 16 weeks in those with type 1 diabetes and signs of retinopathy at the first antenatal appointment. Hypertension and pre-eclampsia are more common in diabetic mothers.

Gestational diabetes mellitus

GDM is defined as glucose intolerance with onset or first recognition during pregnancy. Previously there were no uniformly accepted international standards for the diagnosis of GDM. New evidence has emerged to change practice. The large multinational Hyperglycemia and Pregnancy Outcome (HAPO) study has demonstrated a linear relationship between maternal hyperglycemia and birthweight, with no apparent threshold effect between maternal glycemia and pregnancy outcome. The Australian Carbohydrate Intolerance Study in Pregnant Women (ACHOIS) has established that treatment of GDM with insulin improves pregnancy outcomes (such as birthweight, macrosomia and shoulder dystocia). The International Association of Diabetes and Pregnancy Study Groups (IADPSG) has attempted to achieve an international consensus on screening and diagnosis of gestational diabetes. It recommends a 75 g oral glucose tolerance test (OGTT) for all women who are not known to be diabetic at

24–28 weeks. Gestational diabetes is diagnosed when one or more threshold values are exceeded (fasting $\geq$ 5.1 mmol/L [92 mg/dL], 1-hour $\geq$ 10.0 mmol/L [180 mg/dL], 2-hour $\geq$ 8.5 mmol/L [153 mg/dL]). Other guidelines (for example, those from the Scottish Intercollegiate Guidelines Network [SIGN]) advocate a more selective approach to screening on the basis of risk factors (for example, obesity, a first-degree relative with diabetes, ethnicity, advanced maternal age, previous GDM and a previous macrosomic baby).

Women should be screened for risk factors at booking. In the USA, a two-step approach has been recommended: a 50 g 1-hour glucose challenge being performed at 26–28 weeks followed by a 100 g 3-hour OGTT for those with an abnormal result in the first test. For high-risk women, a one-step approach could be used by proceeding directly to the 100 g 3-hour OGTT. However, at present, the American Diabetes Association is planning to consider adoption of the IADPSG diagnostic criteria. Those with previous GDM should start early self-monitoring of blood glucose or have a 2-hour 75 g OGTT at 16–18 weeks followed by a repeat OGTT at 28 weeks if the first test is normal. In the presence of other risk factors, an OGTT should be undertaken at 24–28 weeks. GDM usually appears after the middle of the second trimester and much of the perinatal morbidity in GDM is associated with the delivery of a large-for-gestational-age baby. The risks associated with GDM are listed in Table 12.2.

Management. Scans to determine fetal growth and abdominal circumference help inform decisions about the need for intensive blood glucose control in GDM. The diagnosis of GDM confers the need to detect maternal hyperglycemia by intensive self-monitoring of blood glucose, preferably by postprandial testing.

All women should receive dietary advice from a dietitian and be encouraged to take physical exercise. Weight loss is recommended for women with a body mass index (BMI) above 27 kg/m^2.

Pharmacological treatment is recommended when fasting blood glucose values exceed 5.3 mmol/L (95 mg/dL) or 2-hour postprandial glucose values exceed 6.7 mmol/L (120 mg/dL). Metformin is now considered acceptable in the treatment of GDM, though it is still not

TABLE 12.2

Risks to women and babies associated with gestational diabetes mellitus

- Fetal macrosomia
- Birth trauma to mother and baby
- Induction of labor or Cesarean section
- Transient neonatal morbidity
- Neonatal hypoglycemia
- Perinatal death

widely used. When glucose targets are not met, and particularly when fetal ultrasound shows incipient fetal macrosomia, insulin therapy should be started. Recent evidence suggests that glibenclamide may also be useful in the treatment of GDM.

Advising women. Women with GDM need to be informed that the condition confers an increased risk of future development of type 2 diabetes and should be strongly advised to reduce this risk postnatally by reducing weight and taking regular exercise. Fasting plasma glucose should be checked at the 6-week postnatal appointment and annually thereafter to check whether the woman has progressed to type 2 diabetes.

Neonatal checks

Neonatal care involves the detection of hypoglycemia, hyperbilirubinemia, respiratory distress, polycythemia and other complications consequent to maternal hyperglycemia during pregnancy.

Babies born to diabetic mothers are at increased risk of developing obesity and diabetes.

Key points – pregnancy and diabetes

- Diabetic pregnancy is associated with fetal morbidity.
- Miscarriage rates are high in diabetic pregnancy.
- The congenital malformation rate is 5.1–9.8%.
- Both growth restriction and growth acceleration may complicate diabetic pregnancy.
- Fetal macrosomia increases the likelihood of birth injury.
- Strict glycemic control improves the outcome of diabetic pregnancy.
- Gestational diabetes mellitus (GDM) is defined as glucose intolerance with onset during pregnancy.
- GDM is becoming increasingly common, particularly in certain ethnic groups.
- Treatment of GDM is associated with improved fetal outcome.

Key references

Crowther CA, Hiller JE, Moss JR et al; Australian Carbohydrate Intolerance Study in Pregnant Women (ACHOIS) Trial Group. Effect of treatment of gestational diabetes mellitus on pregnancy outcomes. *N Engl J Med* 2005;352:2477–86.

The HAPO Study Cooperative Research Group. Hyperglycemia and adverse pregnancy outcomes. *N Engl J Med* 2008;358:1991–2002.

Homko CJ, Reece EA. Insulins and oral hypoglycemic agents in pregnancy. *J Matern Fetal Neonatal Med* 2006;18:1442–5.

Metzger BE, Gabbe SG, Persson B et al. International association of diabetes and pregnancy study groups recommendations on the diagnosis and classification of hyperglycemia in pregnancy. *Diabetes Care* 2010;33:676-82.

Taylor R, Lee C, Kyne-Grzebalski D et al. Clinical outcomes in women with type 1 diabetes. *Obstet Gynecol* 2002;99;537–41.

Useful resources

UK
Diabetes Research and Wellness
Foundation
Tel: +44 (0)23 92 637 808
www.drwf.org.uk

Diabetes UK
Careline: 0845 120 2960
(Mon–Fri, 9.00 AM–5.00 PM)
Tel: +44 (0)20 7424 1000
careline@diabetes.org.uk
www.diabetes.org.uk

Juvenile Diabetes Research
Foundation
Tel: +44 (0)20 7713 2030
info@jdrf.org.uk
www.jdrf.org.uk

National Institute for Health and
Clinical Excellence
Tel: 0845 003 7780
www.nice.org.uk
Diabetes guidelines: www.nice.org.
uk/guidance/index.
jsp?action=byTopic&o=7239#/
search/?reload, accessed 09 May
2012

NHS Diabetes
Tel: +44 (0)191 229 2947
enquiries@diabetes.nhs.uk
www.diabetes.nhs.uk

USA
American Diabetes Association
Tel: 1 800 342 2383
(Mon–Fri, 8.30 AM–8.00 PM)
AskADA@diabetes.org
www.diabetes.org

International
Canadian Diabetes Association
Tel: +1 416 363 3373
info@diabetes.ca
www.diabetes.ca

Diabetes Australia
Infoline: 1300 136 588
Tel: +61 (02) 6232 3800
admin@diabetesaustralia.com.au
www.diabetesaustralia.com.au

European Association for the
Study of Diabetes
Tel: +49 211 758 4690
secretariat@easd.org
www.easd.org

International Diabetes
Federation
Tel: +32 2 538 5511
info@idf.org
www.idf.org

Index